The Pe

I'm Sorry, But Your PERFUME MAKES ME SICK . . .

And So Does Almost Everything Else That Smells

KATHY GLENN

Published by
Bluebird Books
Box 241
Unity, Wisconsin 54488

Printed by

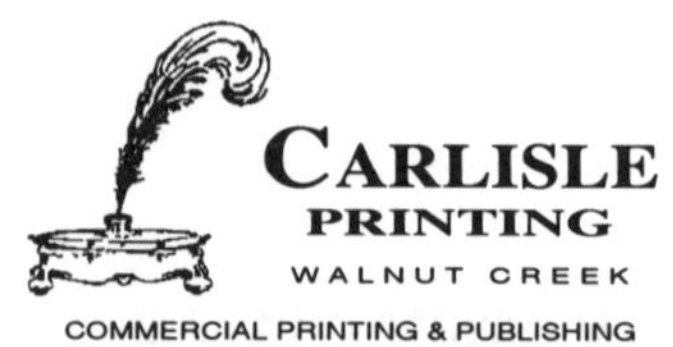

COMMERCIAL PRINTING & PUBLISHING
2727 Press Run Rd. • Sugarcreek, OH 44681

Dedication

This volume is dedicated to my precious husband and to our children, who suffered with me through the fourteen years of seemingly indefensible symptoms detailed herein. They have my most humble gratitude for standing by me when I appeared most unworthy of their support. Nothing but love could have prevented them from abandoning me during those years of turmoil.

It is also dedicated to God, the Creator and Sustainer of all things, Who so graciously sustained me while I went through many experiences that were very strange indeed. His grace was ever sufficient. I take credit only for the failures, for they were all my own.

Disclaimer

The author of this book has undertaken to tell you about her own experience with sensitivity to chemicals in the air. She has also described the route that led, albeit slowly and not altogether completely, to her recovery. Neither she nor the publisher are claiming that the use of a similar regime of supplements and lifestyle changes will cause an identical response to hers in any other individual. Nor are they recommending that you use this book to self diagnose any ailment that you might be experiencing. Similarly, it is not their intention that you use the information to diagnose for anybody else.

There are professionally trained practitioners who do these things. To contact one, see references in the appendix of this book. In the event that any reader should choose to use the information in this book without professional guidance, he is prescribing for himself. He has the constitutional right to do this. However, neither the author nor the publisher accepts any responsibility for his having done so, nor yet for the results that he might obtain, be they good or bad.

Table of Contents

Foreword

Does strong perfume make you dizzy, or Clorox give you a headache? Do cigarette smoke or diesel exhaust make you feel like throwing up? Do insecticides, fresh paint and varnish, cleaning products, scented personal care items, or the detergent aisle in the grocery store fuzz up your thinking or make your chest feel tight? Does a stop at the service station or the dry cleaner's leave you spaced out and anxious, or even irrational?

The above are given as examples only, of course; you might experience different reactions than these. The point is not the exact combination of cause and effect. The point is that if you experience symptoms such as the above when you're exposed to this type of substances, then the time to do something about it is now, before the problem gets worse. For when such a condition reaches its full development, it can become a nightmare. Let me assure you that you never want to go through anything that even begins to approach the horrors I experienced as a direct result of sensitivity to chemicals in the air.

This book is designed to help you avoid those reactions instead of having to escape from their tendrils once they have enmeshed you.

Introduction

One day in 1975, I suddenly found that I couldn't breathe when near the exhaust from a diesel engine. Some time later, I had the same response around insecticides. A few months later, strong perfume caused an identical reaction.

When I described my new problem to our friends, they couldn't understand it. How could there be a connection between not being able to breathe and the presence of chemicals in the air? After all, everyone was exposed to such things, and no one else stopped breathing. They'd never heard of such a thing before.

We hadn't either. So far as we knew, I was the only person in the world who couldn't breathe in the presence of these things. Such weird reactions left us very confused. It was both embarrassing and frustrating to be made ill by a friend's perfume — a fragrance that I'd worn myself until very recently. People have worn perfume since Cleopatra's day. Why should it make me ill?

More than one well-meaning friend indicted my imagination. "It doesn't bother me," they'd say. "Why should it bother you?" I was glad for their sakes that it didn't make them a problem. But I could have handled a little more sympathy, especially as my sensitivities became more and more severe. (By the fall of 1989, I couldn't get my breath within a few seconds of anyone opening an ordinary felt-tip marker anywhere in the house. I was too sensitive to go anywhere, and I couldn't handle visitors in the house unless they had first washed their clothing in fragrance-free detergent and dried it outdoors. Of course they didn't dare to wear any sort of personal care products at all.)

Today, more and more people are reacting negatively to chemicals in the air. "That makes me sick!" they cry in response to exposures that don't affect their "normal" friends.

There are two stages of sensitivity to chemicals. In the above discussion, the victim himself can easily link the symptom with its cause. He inhales smoke and gets a headache, becomes nauseated, or experiences burning eyes and/or airways. Maybe he also feels sick all over, or is unable to breathe.

Such reactions are enough to generate misunderstandings. But the second stage is even more mysterious. In it, the victim experiences a dimension of sensitivity that goes far beyond reactions to things that he or others can smell. He begins to respond negatively to irritants that even the most sensitive of normal noses can't detect. In many cases, his own nose can't detect them either.

Today, literally hundreds of thousands of individuals in the so-called civilized world are suffering many very strange and varied symptoms as a direct result of exposure to chemical concentrations that are low enough to pass undetected.

In the midst of such low levels of exposure, the victim might be aware that he's reacting to something. More often, though, he doesn't realize he's affected. (I soon came to recognize a certain look that would pass between the members of my family just before one or another of them would suggest that it's probably time for us to leave where ever we were at the time. They, not I, had realized that my mental functioning was being negatively affected by something in the environment. They would never have been aware of the presence of an irritant otherwise, but my aberrant behavior had given it—and me—away.)

Because there's no other seemingly logical explanation, such responses are usually ascribed to the imagination or to mental imbalances. "Whatever's wrong with Pete," folks say, "he sure is acting strange."

Such sensitivity is becoming increasingly common. So, of course, are the underlying causes. Fortunately for the victims, public awareness is growing, albeit slowly. Terms such as environmental illness, immune system disregulation, candida overgrowth, chronic fatigue syndrome, and even such simple terms as allergy, are becoming better known. Twenty-five years hence, they'll likely all be a part of our everyday language.

In 1976, however, when I desperately needed understanding and acceptance, only a handful of people anywhere knew that such reactions were genuine physical responses. Very few, in fact, were aware that such reactions could exist. None of them were people whom we knew.

We now know that even those who were aware of such problems at that time knew of only one solution: avoid exposure to the substances that make you ill. Later on, some very astute observers began to filter through the possibilities to determine what actually causes such sensitivities.

A vast array of bodily imbalances are involved. Glandular disturbances, including thyroid deficiency as well as adrenal exhaustion with its resultant hypoglycemia. Candida overgrowth and the multitude of strange imbalances it can create in the body. Immune system disregulation, with the autoimmune, allergic, and various other responses under which it masquerades.

Along with the above, and complicating things further, we find nutrient deficiencies and frequently also the presence of heavy metals in the tissues. We also find body toxicity. This is mainly caused by the incomplete digestion of foods, especially of proteins. Much of this toxicity is associated with the daily consumption of foods to which the individual is actually allergic — and frequently addicted.

All of these irregularities and others similar to them are becoming increasingly common for several reasons. The environment is being contaminated with untold numbers of untested and often unsafe chemicals which are rained upon us not only one at a time, but also in varying combinations that never have been tested for their cumulative effects.

Almost our entire population now faces the results of rampant antibiotic use and abuse over the past fifty years. This is complicated by the effects of other medications, such as birth control pills, that further unbalance the body's ecology.

We also have to consider the perversion of our food — the plethora of so-called junk food (I call it junk foodless) that we've grown to think of as normal fare. We know it's "not good for us," but most of us like it far too well to allow our intellects to overrule our tastebuds.

All these things are against us. Those who have strong constitutions still seem to be coping fairly well. But those who were born with weaker bodies have less resistance, and are breaking down under the onslaught of our unbalanced living. Obviously, I was one of the weak ones.

Do you, or does someone you love, experience unexplainable physical and/or mental symptoms in the presence of obvious levels of chemicals in the air? Then please remember that you are not alone. Tens of thousands of North Americans and Europeans already share your fate. Every one of them sympathizes: their symptoms might not be the same as yours, but their frustrations are certainly similar.

And please do read this book. Just as I did, you might find answers to your bizarre problems. It takes dedication to overcome the underlying imbalances, but it really can be done. I know, for it happened to me. I became far more sensitive than detailed in this introduction, and I've now recovered to a remarkable degree. While not totally well yet, I enjoy life again, and look forward to each new day with anticipation rather than with dread.

So if you experience physical and/or mental symptoms that the medical world can't explain — symptoms for which they want to refer you to a psychiatrist — give a moment to consider the possibility that your problems might be caused by physical imbalances, both in your body and in the environment around you. No amount of counselling will help that.

You need to understand your body. This book is a place to start. The recommended reading in the appendix will give you further valuable information. Take charge of your health by learning all you can and then putting it to practice. There will never be a better time than now to start.

Chapter One

Go Home and Die

My husband and I had consulted numerous doctors over the years, always hoping to find someone who had answers to my strange and varied symptoms—a doctor who knew what to do with a collection of weird manifestations that refused to fit into the description of any known disease. My final medical appointment was in October of 1989.

By this time, my degree of sensitivity to chemicals in the air I breathed (this was my major area of difficulty) had increased to the point where I could not force even very lightly contaminated air to go into my lungs. The air in a doctor's office is certainly contaminated with chemicals.

When we arrived at the clinic, therefore, my husband went into the building and made arrangements with the receptionist to open a window in the room where the doctor would speak with me. She also agreed to notify me when he was ready to see me. Meanwhile, I was to wait on the steps outside until she called me in.

Once summoned inside, I held my breath as I hurried through the waiting room and down the hall. I stood beside the open window in the examining room, thankful that the breeze was blowing inward.

The doctor entered and sat behind his desk. "Your medical findings are negative again," he said slowly. He aligned each finger tip precisely with its counterpart on the other hand as he spoke. "All I can say is, go home and see what happens."

I watched him with a mixture of mild disgust and increasing fascination as he talked, amazed at the degree of detachment he was able to maintain. From intuition as well as from reading, I knew what would come next. When people react strangely, either physically or mentally, to levels of chemicals in the air that don't bother other people, a negative lab result is to be expected.

This failure of the lab to detect any physical abnormality is then taken as proof that the patient's problems are in his head—that what he needs is psychiatric care. Looking back, I can certainly understand why most of our acquaintances had reached that conclusion about me some time ago already. Anyone who behaved as I did had to have some kind of mental problem.

Fortunately for me, my doctor didn't agree. "We know you're desperately ill," he said. "Your symptoms have to have physical causes. But you seem to be on the leading edge of something new. This whole field of allergy to substances in the air is just coming to light. Research is beginning, but no one seems to have any answers yet. In fact, most people in the medical world don't yet accept the possibility that chemicals in the air can make some people acutely ill when they don't bother others at all."

I had already learned by reading that many medical doctors, when they're eyeball-to-eyeball with chemical sensitivity, will diagnose mental involvement and refer the patient to a psychiatrist. Under such treatment, the failure rate approaches 100 percent. These people, even when their symptoms seems to be mostly mental, are physically ill.

Apparently my doctor knew this well. He cleared his throat and went on speaking. "We've already discussed the futility of counseling. Your problems are not in that area. Unfortunately, I have nothing more to offer."

His gaze met mine for a moment before it returned to his finger tips. "I conferred with a clinical ecologist as you requested, hoping she might know of some way to help you. She says you're already doing everything she could suggest. She doesn't dare to test you: a reaction to the test solution could kill you. She says you should continue to avoid the things that make you sick. She expects you'll live for about two more years. If you get trapped in a situation where you're exposed to some chemical your system can't handle, of course, and can't get away, it would be less than two years."

Throughout the entire speech, the doctor maintained the poise of the perfect professional. When this interview was over, he could go on to other patients, some of whom, at least, he could offer hope. For me, he had done the best he knew how. His only remaining option was to dismiss me.

"I'm sorry to be so negative," he said as he stood to signal the end of the interview. "As I already said, you're on the leading edge of something new."

I had no question to ask, no thought to share. Something inside of me knew—had known for what seemed like a lifetime already—that someday this would come: "Go home and die."

A short period of halfhearted grief followed the medical man's pronouncement; a brief lament for the future that would never be. The traveling my hubby and I had talked about doing someday. The grandchildren we had been looking forward to, none of whom were yet born. Growing old together.

My regrets did not last long, however, for I had already suspected that my time on earth would be short. The death warrant issued by the doctor served only to verify my own conclusion, and knowing for sure brought more relief than sorrow.

My easy truce with death was partly because of the perplexing chemical sensitivities and resultant restrictions on my life, and partly because I'd already lived with chronic pain for many years. (More about that later in the story.) I'd been able to cope with the thirty plus years of pain, the twelve years of terrible tiredness, and the ten or more years of really weird mental and physical symptoms no one had an explanation for. But when the chemical sensitivity got suddenly severe late in 1989, I really did come to the threshold of despair. I was desperate for release, and I constantly asked the Lord to take me Home.

Now the doctor's verdict, combined with the clinical ecologist's conclusion that I might live for two more years, provided a welcome prospect of escape. I even hoped they were overly optimistic; that I wouldn't have to live that long.

The Beginning of my Chemical Story

In 1959, thirty years before my chemical sensitivity suddenly became extreme, each student in my high school received a prick of tuberculosis test solution under the skin of his forearm. From among more than twelve hundred students, I had the only positive response.

I didn't have TB, though; the x-ray showed nothing. A false positive, the radiologist explained. At the time of the test, of course, I was so embarrassed by being made to stand apart from the herd that I didn't question what else the welt raised by the test solution might mean. (Who might I have asked who would have known anyhow?)

Many years later, I learned that a false positive on tuberculosis screening is often an indicator of immune system disregulation. And immune system disregulation is a part of the cause of chemical sensitivity.

Looking back, I suppose that this was the first real inkling that my biochemical individuality would someday go berserk. The first indication that the warrior portion of my immune system was flashing red alert when it should have been on hold.

Some of my Earliest Problems

As a child, I didn't know I wasn't normal. People called me lazy. Well, I thought, why shouldn't I prefer to read instead of playing baseball? I was in my middle teens before I realized that not everyone is tired all the time.

My earliest recollections deal with pain. My very early respiratory problems were followed by constant aching in my legs. Both were bad by the time I started school. But growing pains were in fashion at the time, so no one took my complaining seriously. I wasn't taken to a doctor until I couldn't walk.

I had rheumatic fever. This was in 1951, and my doctor had a passion for the then newly discovered antibiotics. Everyone who went to his office got a shot. I was pumped full of penicillin for three months for the fever, receiving it both by injection and by mouth. (It wasn't until about 1987 that I learned about the connection between antibiotics and candida yeast overgrowth—and the relationship of candida overgrowth to chemical sensitivities.)

After three months of penicillin, I was well enough to go back to school. The pain in my legs, however, never went away. Before long, my arms began to ache as well, and soon I hurt all over. I also had a heart murmur from the fever.

Exertion made my discomfort worse, so my life began to revolve around whether or not an activity would generate more pain. I sat on the sidelines a lot of the time—an onlooker nursing my aching limbs and watching the world go by.

When I got into my teens, I tired of being called lazy, and began to do more work in spite of the pain. It got to be a martyr sort of thing; it hurts me something awful, but because it's expected of me, I'll do it anyway.

The doctor said the pain was an aftermath of the rheumatic fever, and that I'd have it for the remainder of my life. About thirty-five years after I'd had the fever, we learned about fibromyalgia and its association with the many other symptoms of chronic fatigue syndrome. I was well into chronic fatigue by the time I learned of its existence.

I was twelve years old when I broke my back, and forty-five when I learned that it had never healed. All that now holds me together in my lower back is muscles, ligaments, and tendons. The bone is completely separated.

I lived with pain from the day of the break—a new kind of pain that was added to the muscle aching—an almost overpowering misery that has often kept me awake into the small hours of the morning. A pain that has prevented me from doing a great many things that others do without a thought. I often wonder now how much the stress of that constant misery has contributed to the overall breakdown of my health.

After my back had hurt for many years, I learned that people who are sensitive to chemicals in the air they breathe are quite likely to experience extra discomfort from old injuries. The chemicals get into their circulation, and from there settle into the area of weakness created by the injury.

My Early Love Affair with DDT

Because it is important to the story and yet doesn't seem to fit conveniently anywhere, I want to discuss the history of my DDT exposure here. First, for those who don't recognize the acronym, DDT refers to diethyl-diphenol-trichloroethane. This insecticide first came on the market in 1939, but the danger it posed to humans was not well understood until much later. (It was not banned for general use in the United States until 1972.)

My passion for the smell of the substance goes back further than I remember. We moved into a log house in 1948, when I was three. We soon found out that the bedbugs had gotten there first. Mother sprinkled DDT powder into the cracks between the logs as well as into the tufts at the edges of the mattresses every few weeks for the four or five years we lived there. It kept the bugs at bay, though they were never totally eliminated.

I loved the smell of this potent insecticide, and would lie in bed inhaling lungful after lungful every time it was used. When I got a little older, I discovered that I could reach the bag of it on the pantry shelf. I would shake the bag, then undo the string that held it shut and inhale the dust. No one worried about it at the time. This was before anyone knew it could harm anything but bugs.

Several doctors have since told me that the insecticide has

permanently damaged my liver. Since the liver is the organ that must detoxify poisons as they enter the body, its damaged condition probably explains my severe sensitivity to chemicals. They get from the lungs to the blood stream, then because the liver doesn't have the power to detoxify them, they continue to circulate through both my body and my brain, upsetting many delicately balanced systems including mental functioning.

The fact that insecticides cause liver damage also helps to explain why chemical sensitivity has become much more widespread in the general population than it used to be. More and more such toxic substances are entering the environment as the years go by. (The effects of candida yeast overgrowth, mainly caused by antibiotics and birth control pills, will be discussed later in the book.)

Chapter Two

An Effort to Begin at the Beginning

I'm writing the final draft of this book in 1996. When sensitivity to chemicals is mentioned today, almost anyone will acknowledge that either he or someone he knows has some degree of either physical or mental reaction when exposed to any noticeable concentration of chemicals in the air.

This awareness that inhaled chemicals can cause problems has increased considerably during the past ten years. Twenty years ago, however, when my chemical intolerance first became obvious to me and my husband, no one we met had ever heard of anyone being made acutely ill by such things as diesel fumes, insecticides, cigarette smoke, or perfume in the air they breathed. The idea seemed impossible to everyone, ourselves included.

In 1975, diesel fumes, insecticides, and strong perfumes were the only chemicals that made me feel acutely ill. If the concentration in the air was great enough, I couldn't breathe. If it was low enough that it didn't stop my respiration, it would give me a headache and muddle up my brain.

In retrospect, we know that these lower concentrations were

already making problems for me much earlier. At that point, however, we didn't make the association. As far back as 1970, trips to town, church, or social functions were almost always followed by a headache and an overall blah feeling that would last for several hours. Traveling brought the same symptoms. So did sleeping with my head on a foam pillow.

Mondays were usually bad days. Looking back, we suppose it was because I did the laundry that day, using a wringer washer and lots of soap and Clorox. Some days, I'd have a bad time for what looked to us like no reason at all.

We finally decided that my problems were induced by stress. The possibility of chemical involvement never occurred to us until I found myself unable to breathe in the presence of diesel exhaust. Then we began to wonder whether more of my strange symptoms might be traceable to the presence of chemicals in the air.

By that point, I'd done some reading about hypoglycemia (low blood sugar) as well. Because some of my symptoms seemed to fit with what I read, we had the medical testing done. The six hour glucose tolerance test confirmed our suspicion: I had serious irregularities in that area. When we learned that for sure, we added hypoglycemia to the stress factor, and blamed the combination for the many strange symptoms, both mental and physical, that I was experiencing at the time.

Hypoglycemia History

The fifth hour reading on my six hour glucose tolerance test was thirty-five. A normal fasting reading is ninety to one hundred. A working level is one hundred ten to one hundred thirty. Most people become unconscious when it drops to thirty-five. The downward spiral ends somewhere around ten; the person dies.

During the test, I experienced several of the symptoms that had been bothering me. Spiralling black dots gyrated before my eyes, and flashes of brilliant light were mixed among them. I felt as though I was walking on a cushion of air about three inches thick, and I couldn't get my feet to go all the way to the floor because it was in the way.

I perceived my intellect as being detached from my body—the mental disconnected from the physical. I sensed a vague sort of identification with my seemingly disembodied intelligence, which I perceived as hovering a few inches below the ceiling in a corner of the room. It was getting a big joke out of watching the physical part of me make a fool of itself.

At the time, of course, we blamed all these eerie symptoms on the low levels of glucose circulating in my blood stream. Looking back, we wonder whether more might have been involved.

I had the test done at the lab in a hospital, and I stayed inside the building for the entire seven hours. The chemical content of hospital air is bad to say the least, even in the best of circumstances. But added to that was the fact that this particular hospital had just been built. I was in the presence of a plethora of chemicals that outgas from new building materials.

How many of my strange reactions that day were actually from the low sugar levels and how many were from the chemicals in the air I breathed all day? I suppose we'll never know. But even today, more than twenty years later, exposure to low levels of chemicals in the air—levels that are too low to stop my breathing—will make me nauseated and give me a headache. They may also bring on the feeling of disconnectedness. Sometimes, I feel as though I'm floating in the air, or that my intellect is floating somewhere above my body.

The doctor who ordered the test for me didn't believe in hypoglycemia. When the results came back, however, he admitted that I had a real problem. He also acknowledged that he didn't have a clue as to what could be done to help me.

"You might consult a nutritionist," he suggested. "The nurse can set up an appointment for you in the city if you wish."

But my husband was working at semivoluntary service at the time, supporting me and the family on minimum wage. We had no money for two-hundred mile trips to the city, let alone a nutritionist's fees.

I had already read Dr. Carlton Fredericks' book Low Blood Sugar and You. That's where we had picked up the idea that my symptoms might be caused by low blood sugar. Now I reread the book, and I muddled along by myself the best I could.

Taming the Sugar Monster

Table sugar is sucrose. Fruit contains fructose. Honey is, according to World Book, made up of levulose and dextrose. Milk sugar is lactose. Corn syrup combines maltose and dextrose.

Body sugar (blood sugar) is glucose. These sugars are all similar, and the others are easily converted to glucose, the form used by the body. When the blood sugar levels are low, therefore, any of the above will satisfy the craving for sugar. But the body knows that the more readily available forms, such as honey and table sugar, will satisfy the craving more rapidly than the more slowly digested sources of sugar such as vegetables and whole grains will.

My body was often low on glucose; we knew that for sure after I had the glucose tolerance test. Therefore, I craved sugar. So the taming of the sugar monster became very necessary. Dr. Fredericks' book helped us to get a handle on the problem, certainly. But the sugar monster was actually far from tamed for many years.

It is beyond the scope of this book to describe the symptoms and treatment of low blood sugar. Please see the Appendix for a list of books on the subject.

I had craved (and therefore had eaten) huge amounts of sugar for most of my life. The hypoglycemia diagnosis finally convinced me that if I continued to do so, sugar would some day destroy me. But the Lord knew how desperately I craved it, especially at three in the afternoon.

My husband, too, realized that this was more than just a casual desire for something sweet. I was literally driven by a desperate need. He therefore decided that we would purge our house of sugar and everything made from it. Had he not, I seriously doubt that I could have stuck to the sugar-free diet that was absolutely necessary to bring the hypoglycemia under control.

For those readers who aren't aware of the relationship between sugar and low levels of blood sugar, here's a supersimplified explanation: eating sugar does raise the blood sugar level temporarily, but the raised level calls forth insulin, and then the level plummets lower than before the sugar was consumed.

The first symptom of low blood sugar levels is often hunger—for something sweet. I had baked something sweet almost every day for years already. But by the time the sugar urge hit again—and it always did in the middle of the afternoon—yesterday's goodies were long gone. I had eaten the last of them within two hours of making them.

I told myself that I made the cookies for my family. But inside I knew differently. I was very overweight, and knew that sweet things made it worse. But the sugar craving overrode my desire to be slim. Every day after I'd eaten my cookies, I'd tell myself, "Tomorrow I'll start to diet."

The sugar tolerance test had proved my inability to handle sweets; that gave more incentive to quit. The weird reactions I had during the test paralleled some of my uncanny everyday symptoms, leading us to conclude that all my strange problems were caused by low blood sugar levels.

So I stuck to Dr. Fredericks' food guidelines. I found, though, that if I was to avoid the desperate sugar cravings, I had to eat more often than he recommended. I finally settled on every two hours all day and every three hours all night. I still craved sweets, but as long as I followed my self-imposed schedule, I could maintain a reasonable control over the sugar monster.

Nevertheless, hypoglycemia remained a major factor in my life for many more years. The moment I went off the diet schedule, I was back in trouble. Not until 1990, when I finally learned how to treat my underlying adrenal exhaustion, did the craving for sugar finally go away. (That information is given later in this book.)

The negative effects I experienced when I did occasionally eat sugar during the intervening years got worse as time went on. Soon just one cookie brought enough reaction to leave me flat on the floor, unable to move or make the least sound for about twenty minutes.

We often wondered during those years why I couldn't overcome the craving for sugar. Then in 1979, my mother told me that as a young child I sleepwalked to the kitchen night after night, about two or three o'clock in the morning. Once there, I ate—and if there were sweets available, that's what I'd have. (Blood sugar levels are usually at their lowest at that time, even in normal people.) When Mother told me about my eating in my sleep, I finally understood why the urge for sweets pervaded my entire life.

Chapter Three

My Earliest Problems with Building Materials

In the summer of 1975, we installed quite an area of new paneling and cushioned vinyl flooring in our house. We also did some painting. At this point, the only connection we had yet made between chemicals and my health was that in the presence of insecticides or strong diesel fumes, I couldn't breathe.

Once the new building materials were in place, my problems began to increase. At the time, we never dreamed that there might be any connection between the deterioration in my health and the building supplies that we had used. We didn't learn about that until twelve years later.

Then the Suspended Animation Spells

I call the spells I started to get about that time suspended animation because I can think of no better name. At first, they came only when I was under stress. Later on, they failed to follow a pattern.

They start with a strange swooning sensation—a feeling

that my body, including my bones, is about to turn to jelly. Within a few seconds, I'm prostrate, unable to move or make the least sound. Usually all I have time to do is get myself onto the floor before I fall.

The spell lasts for about twenty minutes. Then my strength gradually returns. After a while, I can get up and begin to move around. Total recovery takes several hours, during which time I'm often, though not always, cold. My speech is very labored for a while after a spell; it takes an incredible amount of effort to talk.

The suspended animation spells wear me out physically and emotionally, dragging me down more effectively than heavy physical work does. They have never followed any discernible pattern. Late in the 1970s, when they were at their worse, I'd sometimes have several in a day. At other times, I could go for several weeks without any.

No doctor I've described these spells to has ever heard of anything quite like them. One doctor suggested a strange form of epileptic seizure, but further investigation failed to bear out that theory. At the time they were at their worst, we learned that I had hypoglycemia (low blood sugar), and from some reading I did then, I came to blame the spells on that. However, there are aspects of them that I now know don't fit into hypoglycemia either. Pain, for example, is magnified.

It isn't unusual, given the condition of my back, for me to land on the floor in a position that isn't comfortable. I can neither move nor ask to be moved. The discomfort can became intense. It's a strange combination of sensations to already be immobile and then to feel as though I might pass out because of the pain in my back.

My sense of touch becomes acute. For example, a fly walking on my face will cause exquisite itching, but I can't do anything about it—not even ask someone to shoo it off.

My hearing is fine. I know what is being said, and know the answers to questions people are asking about me, and so on. I even know that given twenty minutes, I'll be able to get up again. I know exactly where I am and what has happened.

In some ways, my mind seems clearer than at other times.

For those who might suspect me of using drugs, the answer is that people who are sensitive to chemicals don't take foolish risks: even ordinary pain medications could increase my sensitivity to chemicals, and so I don't use them in spite of the chronic discomfort I experience.

If anyone who reads this has ever had a series of similar episodes, I'd encourage you to contact me through the publisher of this book. I'd like to know about your experience. So far, I've never met anyone whose experiences in this area have come anywhere near to paralleling these suspended animation spells.

Brand-New, Superinsulated House

The deterioration in my health following the renovations we made in our house in the summer of 1975 had failed to alert us to the dangers of brand new building materials. I suppose it's not much wonder we didn't get the point: at this time, only a very few people anywhere knew about the connection between the chemicals outgassed into the air by such substances and the strange new maladies some people were experiencing. The people who did respond negatively to these materials were generally thought to have mental problems, and no connection was made to the real cause of the difficulty.

Because we hadn't made any such connection, in the fall of 1977 we moved into a brand-new, superinsulated house. My health got worse immediately, but once again, we hadn't a clue why. We built that house in 1977, and not until 1987, ten years after we built it and seven years after we sold it, did we learn of the probable connection between the new, superinsulated structure and my ever increasing difficulties.

In 1987, I had cancer, and it was the naturopath whom we consulted then that first told us about the dangers inherent in these very tightly built structures. The danger is especially great when there isn't adequate ventilation. Such buildings, he told us, sometimes cause trouble for even apparently healthy individuals. How much more likely, then, is it that they might make problems for those who, like myself, already suffer from compromised resistance?

We knew nothing of this when we built the house, of course. At the time, superinsulated construction was being touted by the experts as a wonderful means of energy conservation. It is. But almost no one then understood the negative effects such buildings could exert on one's health. Today, almost everyone has heard of the sick building syndrome—though even after the proof is in, some die-hard skeptics still refuse to believe that anyone could be made ill by exposure to the fumes from building materials.

We chose superinsulated construction primarily because we were living in a climate where the summers were very hot, and I minded the heat very much. So we planned to keep the windows open at night and then close them early in the morning, thus keeping the cool night air indoors during the daytime. I stayed indoors, of course, to keep myself cool.

Various health problems escalated quickly for me once we moved into the new house. Most of the symptoms were such that they were considered to be mental in origin. The various forms of disperception that I've suffered ever since to one degree or another became a real trial to me soon after we moved into the new dwelling.

Of course we tried to find something to blame for my strange symptoms. By this point, we had known for some time already that I was suffering from low blood sugar (hypoglycemia). Because we didn't know of anything else that might be causing my problems, we blamed everything, no matter how weird it was, on the blood sugar disregulation. It was the only culprit we knew of.

Looking back now, and knowing how carefully I adhered to the hypoglycemia diet, we realize that we should have suspected something further amiss. But on the other hand, what might we have suspected? The sick building syndrome hadn't yet been discovered, and no one we ever met had heard anything about the possibility of chemicals in the air leading to physical or mental problems.

We had used an abundance of no-no materials in the construction of the house, of course. The particleboard subfloors were loaded with glues and formaldehyde. So was the ceiling tile, all twenty-eight hundred square feet of it. New carpets and underpadding as well as cushioned vinyl flooring contributed their load of pollutants too, including an abundance of formaldehyde. Vinyl wallpaper and water-base paint on the walls added more of the same. Even the kitchen cabinets were made of particleboard.

Overall, we had created a chemical soup of a very high order indeed, but we didn't realize what we had done. I spent almost all of my time immersed in it to the hilt. With the problems I already had before we moved in, I sometimes wonder how I stayed alive.

To make the effects of the chemicals worse than they might otherwise have been, we moved into the house before it was nearly finished, and did the painting and varnishing, wallpapering and floor covering, after we were living in the building. Just to make things worse, it was November. We had gone to great effort and expense to make a superinsulated dwelling that wouldn't require much heating fuel. Why would we now want to open the windows and thus waste heat? So we did the interior finishing with what we now know was grossly inadequate ventilation.

I felt my energy level dropping during the first months in the new house, and as I noted earlier, my weird symptoms increased dramatically. But we were busy trying to get the house finished, so I forced myself to keep going.

The following spring, however, the day came when I couldn't muster the strength to carry on. At thirty-one years old, I had accumulated too great a load of stressors on my system. I collapsed. After about two weeks in bed, I began to move around inside the house a little.

It was now June, and with the hot weather coming on, we once again kept the windows closed all day. I had just started to get on my feet a little when I came down with an unusual form of pneumonia.

Pneumonia and Afterward

The doctor x-rayed my lungs, found they were already what he designated as one-fourth full, and put me on penicillin for a week. When I went back, he x-rayed me again and doubled the dose. A week after that, he changed my medication to Keflex, and at the end of that week he doubled the dose of it. The pneumonia hadn't budged except to get worse.

At this point he took a culture. The lab ran it with thirteen different antibiotics, only one of which, Carbenicillin, was able to even slow it down. I spent another week or so in the recliner day and night (I couldn't breathe lying down) before the pneumonia started to clear.

When I was finally able to be up, I was desperately tired all the time, even though for almost two months I hadn't done anything but rest. A pervasive weariness had overtaken me—an exhaustion that no amount of sleep could relieve and from which there seemed to be no means of escape.

I complained of it to my doctor, and he said, "My dear woman! You've had a million antibiotics. What else could you expect?"

When questioned, however, he admitted that he didn't know why people who receive large amounts of antibiotics often feel tired afterward, some of them for the remainder of their lives. Ten years later, we learned about candida yeast overgrowth and how it is made worse by antibiotics. Only then did my years of tiredness make sense. (See chapter five for an explanation of the relationship between antibiotic use and candida overgrowth.)

Time Lapses

I'd been having the suspended animation spells quite a while before the time lapses began. Once again, as with the suspended animation, the terminology might not be scientifically accurate. It's just the best name I can think of for what happens.

These time lapses differ entirely from ordinary forgetfulness. I know; I experience both. I don't know I'm in a time lapse until I suddenly feel as though I'm getting awake. I'm then unable to recall anything that has happened during the preceding fifteen or twenty minutes.

For example, I might come out of a time lapse when we're partway through a meal. I will have absolutely no recollection of finishing cooking the food or bringing it to the table. Nor will I remember that someone led in prayer or that we passed the dishes of food and served our plates from them. Even having eaten part of the meal seems impossible; I simply don't remember. It's as though I'd been asleep during the entire procedure. Those twenty minutes are blank, and never come back.

My family insists that I act quite normal during these lapses: I carry on conversations, give directions where appropriate, and so on. Had I not told on myself, they wouldn't have suspected that anything was amiss.

During the suspended animation spells, on the other hand, I'm aware of what is happening and I remember it all afterward. But during the actual spell I'm absolutely unable to move or communicate, so everyone who sees me is very much aware that something is wrong.

Though the time lapses were much more common while we lived in the brand-new, superinsulated house, I still get them occasionally. When they come, I find them emotionally trying, just as I always have. Such weird things never happen to normal people. When I do get one now, I don't mention it to anyone. Why should I deliberately draw attention to something weird?

Coming out of one feels just like waking up. It's rather ironic, for since the initial lapse, I've never been aware of waking from actual sleep. I don't know whether or not I've slept until I check the time. Other than at the end of a memory lapse, I've never known the sensation of waking up for nineteen years.

Consistently Inconsistent

By the time we moved into the superinsulated house, our

children's ages ranged from four to thirteen. The older girls were now taking most of the responsibility for the housework as well as overseeing the younger children.

I knew that I couldn't handle their noise, even when they tried very hard to be quiet. And I knew that I wasn't as patient with them as I should have been, even though I was depending on the Lord for the grace I needed to nurture them for Him. But not until the following incident did I realize at least to some degree how hard I was making life for them.

It's still hard for me to even think about this, much less to discuss it. But I think it has a place in the story—perhaps other mothers are suffering as I was, and could benefit from it.

I had found one of our sons doing something that I felt for his own good he must be punished for, and I gave him a spanking. A few minutes later, our oldest daughter came to me and said, "Mother, I'm sure you don't remember, but I thought maybe I should tell you that just about ten minutes before you spanked him for doing that, you had sent him to do exactly what he was doing."

I found it impossible to believe what she said. There was absolutely not a particle of sense in the idea. I'd never have told him to do that, I knew.

So I asked another of our daughters if she knew anything about it.

"Yes," she answered. "You often say something and then change your mind. I don't think you remember, though, so I don't think it's your fault."

That unbelievable insight came from an eleven year old.

My husband and I have discussed this aspect of my illness several times since I'm well. His comment: "The only consistent thing about your behavior was its inconsistency. We simply never knew what to expect. About all we could count on was that we couldn't count on anything."

My family lived with that inconsistency for at least a dozen years, off and on. The degree of unpredictability depended on the total load on my system at the time. The more stressors, the less consistent I'd be. We didn't understand that, of course, until after I was on my way to recovery.

Occasionally, when I'm trying too hard to get things done and not getting enough rest, it still shows up. But at least I know enough to believe it when someone says to me, "Now you say red geraniums are your favorite flowers. Yesterday you told the lady at the other greenhouse we visited that your number one choice was pink carnations."

But at least I'm no longer consistently inconsistent.

Maladjusted Thermostat

Some of the things I want to discuss in this book don't seem to fit in at any particular place in the narrative. One of these is my maladjusted thermostat.

I had experienced poor tolerance to hot weather before the pneumonia already. Heat levels in which other people were comfortable left me too warm—sometimes far too warm. My comfort range was about fifty to sixty degrees.

When the pneumonia was over, my tolerance had nose-dived until anything above seventy-five degrees left me literally prostrate from the heat. This particular peculiarity kept several doctors from ordering a thyroid function test for me, even when I begged to have it done. People with low thyroids are supposed to be cold, not hot. Just recently, we learned that sometimes if both thyroid and adrenal functions are under par, the person with the problems may be hot instead of cold. (See the section on Adrenal Rebuilding in this book for more information on the adrenal glands.)

So as it turned out, my being hot instead of cold was just one more example of a mix-up in symptoms that was generated by imbalances in my body rather than by my imagination. When several body systems are out of kilter at the same time, it's truly amazing what an assortment of symptoms can be produced.

Chapter Four

Problems with Sound and Space

When the time lapses began, I also started to experience disperceptions with sound and space. In the spatial problem, the walls, floor, and ceiling of the room I'm in all seem to be moving toward me. Slowly but steadily, they come closer and closer, until even in a large room I perceive myself to be in a cubicle about the size of a telephone booth but with a lower ceiling.

I can set everything back to rights by closing my eyes for a few seconds, but as soon as I open them again, the room begins to shrink. Only by closing them for an hour or longer can I get everything to stay in its proper perspective.

I seldom experience this particular problem anymore, and when I do, it's much less intense than it was in the superinsulated house. There, it was very common indeed.

The distortion of sound is even more irritating than the room-shrinking phenomenon is. The sound disperception has stayed with me longer and more consistently too. Its most frustrating aspect is the distortion of music. I've always thoroughly enjoyed our congregational singing at church. But when the disperception began, I found I could no longer trust the singing. Sometimes it sounded exactly like it should, and sometimes the lovely harmony seemed to disintegrate into a chaos of metallic grating and grinding; a swirl of unearthly screeches, moans, and howls—the type of noises one might expect to emanate from the Pit, but which certainly don't belong on earth, and least of all in church.

To get rid of the horrible racket, I'd have to get as far from it as I could, which meant going outside. Sometimes after I came back indoors, the next song would sound all right, and sometimes the nerve-rending discordance would recur.

This distortion of sound wasn't constant. It came at intervals only, albeit with no discernible pattern. In contrast, the volume of sound always seemed louder than it really was. Moreover, the louder a sound actually was, the more likely it was to go out of focus in my brain. This is still the case. Not long ago, a baby's loud crying sent my body into an overall panic: my heart raced and pounded, I broke out into a sweat, and I felt as though my brain was about to explode. What happened to my blood pressure? I'd love to know!

Skin Troubles

Many people who have allergic reactions break out in a rash. I never did. I've often wished I could—that great purple welts would pop out on my skin the moment I was exposed to anything that made me feel ill. (Even then, though, would the skeptics believe I wasn't just putting it on?)

In spite of the fact that nothing anyone could see ever happened to my skin, the invisible misery was very real. The crawling sensations started several years before the snowballing began in the fall of 1989, and grew worse then. Soon after the snowballing got under way, contact with any fabric but cotton or other totally natural substances left me feeling as if a million maggots were crawling on my skin.

My legs became especially sensitive, and ever since, even pure cotton stockings make me miserable. When the crawling sensation was at its worst, I'd often have to get up in the middle of the night and sit with nothing but air in touch with my legs for half an hour. After that, I could usually go back to bed and sleep.

Besides the crawling sensation, I developed burning patches on my body. These began when we moved into the superinsulated house. They range in size from the diameter of a teacup to that of a dinner plate. They come and go at random. For quite a while, it seemed, they mostly came. Sometimes I had four or five of them at once. Some of them last only a few days; others stay for years. The one on the bottom of my left foot began about eight years ago, and hasn't let up since. They feel like a bad sunburn. The warmer the surroundings, the more they burn.

Petrochemical Poisoning

Some authorities on the subject of chemical sensitivity think that the problems people like me experience with fabrics trace to the petrochemicals from which polyesters and other synthetics are made. It seems to be a logical conclusion, for petrochemicals in any form — solid, liquid, or vapor — have made me sick for more than twenty years. With the least exposure, I feel as if there's a noose around my neck. The aura of a service station still bothers me. It used to make me feel as though an elephant was sitting on my chest. Exhaust would do the same. Even now, it bothers me on a hot day in heavy traffic.

Some people are more sensitive to petrochemicals than I was at any time. But there are others who think they have a serious problem with exhaust fumes, for example, whose stories fail to impress me. They stand there breathing in the fumes while they tell me how ill it makes them. If it did to them what it does to me, they'd move!

Oh, To Sleep!

I don't remember whether the sleeplessness that wasn't caused by pain began before we moved into the superinsulated house or not. I do know that from the age of twelve, when my back was broken, onward. I often didn't sleep because of pain. It would be two or three in the morning before I'd finally drop into exhausted slumber.

I do know that once we were in the new house, I would often be awake for many hours just because I couldn't drop off. Even if I wasn't in pain, and even if I felt relaxed, sleep simply would not come . I'd count the quarter hours by the chime clock in the living room downstairs.

After a while, the chime clock stopped working, but for some reason I still knew within five minutes what time it was all during the night. This even continued after I could sleep again. I'd wake up and I'd know without looking at the clock almost the exact time. This gave me such an eerie feeling that I began to pray for the Lord to take it away from me, and He did. Now I have to check the clock when I want to know the time.

I had several periods of sleep problems throughout the years. Looking back, I know that mostly they centered around the times when I was in settings that had more chemicals in the air. I still have problems getting to sleep on Sunday evenings if we've been to church both morning and evening. I suppose there's just too much buildup of perfume, aftershave, deodorants, and so in my system. After a couple of hours for my body to detoxify, I go to sleep.

Seemingly Unrelated Terrors

Many of the trials I experienced during the years of my most intense reactions would seem to bear no discernible connection to chemical exposure. Nevertheless, those bizarre symptoms improved later on, and the change was in direct proportion to the decrease in my overall sensitivity to chemicals.

Terrors with no basis in fact hounded me for years. That they were phobias only, didn't make them any less real at the time.

The most persistent and most distressing of these seemingly foolish phobias was my dread of reptiles. What if I'd step on a snake? The fear of them dogged my every step for years. I lived with a pervasive dread. Even in the wintertime, I couldn't force myself to get out of bed during the night until I had turned on the light and checked the floor for snakes. I was constantly on the alert for them during the day as well.

I dreamed of them so frequently that I dreaded going to bed. Great, hideous monsters, most of them with two heads, writhed and slithered through my nights. They never actually touched me, but often they managed to come distressingly close. The very thought of kneeling with eyes shut to pray became more than I could endure. What if there were a snake beneath the bed?

Much of the little energy my body was able to muster in those years was wasted watching for snakes that were never there. I didn't tell anyone about them, of course. Why would I have? I was weird enough without adding something like that.

Was there a direct relationship between such phobias and the causes of my sensitivity to chemicals? What about a possible connection with some of my other problems? We think there was, for as the allergic reactions later decreased, not only did my waking fears melt away, but I didn't dream about reptiles anymore. No spiritual or emotional adjustments were made in my life to accomplish the improvement. I didn't even realize that the phobias were fading until they were almost gone.

Now, if I dream of snakes, I know I've been playing too many games with my health-maintenance program. It's time to tighten up my supplement schedule and to stay further from chemicals.

Natural Irritants

Of all the substances that ever made me ill, marsh gas came as the most genuine surprise. One hot summer day in 1985, I found I couldn't get my breath while driving through a swamp. My husband began to take alternative routes in order to avoid the longer marshy areas in summer.

With the first swamp gas encounter, I really did wonder if my brain had slipped a cog. Later, I learned that swamp gas is chemically similar to propane, and it had made me sick for years already. I also learned that other people who are sensitive to chemicals have problems with swamps during the summertime.

Soon after swamp gas began to make trouble, pine and cedar lumber also started to affect my breathing. The newer the lumber was, the worse problem it made. As it aged, it made less difficulty for me, though it still tightened my chest even if well aged.

The foliage of both pine and cedar began to affect my chest also. So did spruce. I couldn't go for a walk in the woods where these species grew; even in winter they made my chest too tight.

Given the degree to which my system had gone off key by this time, I suppose it's not much wonder that the doctors sent me home to die. They knew how real my problems were; they assured me of that. But they also knew that they had nothing for my healing. Sensitivity to chemicals in the air was too new a field, and hardly any of the answers were yet in.

Why Do I Tell You These Things?

I realize that some of the people who read this will take the liberty to decide for themselves how much of it to believe and how much to think I invented on purpose to impress my audience. Given the strangeness of my experiences, I guess I understand that. It hasn't been any fun to be this weird.

I don't enjoy recounting these experiences, either the parts from which I have now recovered or those aspects that even now bother me sometimes. No one wants to be that different. It would have been much easier to remain silent.

But I know there are other sufferers out there—people who sincerely believe that with the sort of symptoms they have, they must surely be alone. People who seriously doubt their own sanity. People who have no inkling that their strange physical, emotional, and mental irregularities could be caused by otherwise undetectable levels of chemicals in the air they're breathing every day. They've given up all hope of being normal.

There are literally thousands of these people scattered across the continent. My earnest desire for each of them is that they or some of their friends might find this little volume and from it might gain the information and courage they need to find their way back to at least some degree of wellness.

We offer no magic; there aren't any easy solutions to these problems. But there is hope, though one has to go outside of the orthodox medical world to find it. They simply do not have the answers because they aren't asking the right questions. We only find the things we're looking for.

I feel blessed today to be able to say that perhaps seventy-five percent of my health has been restored. The route to health wasn't an easy one. Body cleansing is a messy business. Dietary adjustments are sometimes hard to make. Nutrient balancing and glandular modulation require consistent, conscientious effort and the swallowing of a lot of pills. Gandida control can make you feel a whole lot worse before you start to improve.

My wish is that if you're suffering from anything like I was, you'll be able to find a knowledgeable and honest nutrition counselor near you who can direct you to use all of the above therapies together. With this kind of help, you might be able to experience a degree of recovery that you've long since dismissed as impossible to attain. I certainly have, and I thank the Lord for the gains.

Chapter Five

Could Candida be Involved?

I had read an occasional article about candida albicans overgrowth over the years, and had decided I didn't have it. The authorities all said it started in the female organs, and I'd never had a yeast infection in my life. Therefore, I hadn't paid much attention to information on the subject.

So when we got Dr. William Crook's book The Yeast Connection early in 1987, we still knew very little about candida overgrowth. By this time I was well into the jungle of chemical sensitivity. I hadn't been able to read a newspaper for over a year; I couldn't get the stinking printer's ink far enough from my nose and still have the paper close enough to my eyes to read it.

The ink from the newly printed volume of The Yeast Connection strangled me whenever I opened it. I had to prop it open in a remote corner of the house for several hours before I could read each spread. Then it had to go back to the airing process again. I read the entire volume two pages at a time.

I recognized myself in many of the examples the author cited. Therefore I felt very fortunate to be able to locate a doctor who treated candida overgrowth with nystatin, the drug that was highly recommended in Dr. Crook's book. I was eager to begin nystatin treatment.

What is Candida?

The healthy human colon is home to more than three hundred species of organisms, most of them microscopic in size. Among them is candida albicans. Scientists have yet to discover any useful purpose for this yeast aside from its part in helping to decompose the body once the host (you) is dead.

The various species of organisms in the colon act as checks and balances for each other; in the normal colon, a healthy balance is maintained between the various species. Therefore, candida never becomes a problem unless this natural balance is compromised in some manner. When the balance gets out of proportion, the candida can become a raging monster.

The most common cause of imbalance is the use of antibiotics, which kill every organism that comes in their way unless it has built-in resistance to them. Unfortunately for us humans, candida yeast is very resistant to antibiotics, while acidophilus and bifidobacteria, the organisms responsible to keep candida under control, are very easily killed by antibiotics. When this kill-off happens, then candida can become a rampaging monster, not only in the colon but throughout the entire body.

Other factors also initiate and promote the overgrowth of candida yeast. Among them are the following: the use of steroids, including prednisone and birth control pills; high consumption of sugar, honey, syrups, and other refined carbohydrates; the use of foods made from refined grains such as white rice and white bread; a depressed immune system from whatever cause; and severe stress of any kind, including frequent pregnancies.

Some Common Symptoms of Candida

Candida is often called the great imitator, for its symptoms overlap with those of many other illnesses. It's often difficult to sort out exactly what is causing health problems anyhow, and this characteristic of candida makes it even harder yet. Moreover, there still doesn't seem to be a reliable lab test, for candida is a normal inhabitant of the body even when it's healthy. The problems come when there's an overgrowth.

Some of the more common symptoms are: tiredness not relieved by what ought to be enough sleep; a bloated feeling after eating, especially if you've had a lot of sweets or starches or fruit; and mental fogginess or disorientation (often referred to as spaciness). This last symptom includes both the failure of logic and short-term memory and the strange sensation that you are somehow detached from your real self—a very eerie feeling, to say the least.

Secondary symptoms include a literal host of varied problems, many of them overlapping with other physical imbalances in the system. Included here are: a white coating on the tongue and/or a bad taste in the mouth; thrush mouth, and in babies diaper rash that won't go away; intolerance to chemicals in the air and/or in food; poor digestion; diarrhea, constipation, or alternation between the two; food cravings, especially for sweets or starches; urinary tract infections; and a feeling of being disoriented or almost drunk at times in spite of not having taken alcohol.

If the above two sections give you reason to suspect that you have candida problems, I strongly encourage you to go to the library or the bookstore and get the books listed in the appendix of this book under the candida heading.

My Personal Candida Invasion

I had been given antibiotics many times in my life, starting with three months of wall-to-wall penicillin for rheumatic fever when I was seven.

Because the fever had left me with heart valve damage, I had to use massive amounts of antibiotics every time I needed dental work from then on. While we were having our family, I needed frequent fillings, for I hadn't yet learned how to supplement my diet to prevent cavities from forming.

During those years also I had repeated urinary tract infections, and each one meant another round of antibiotics. (I later learned that taking twenty-five milligrams of zinc a day often helps to prevent them, and I haven't had a urinary problem since I started to take it eighteen years ago.)

The antibiotic-resistant pneumonia in the summer of 1978 was the proverbial final straw. All those weeks of antibiotics, a lot of the time on double doses, were followed by a terrible tiredness—a weariness that words can not describe.

The candida came in spite of the fact that I'd been completely off of sugar for a couple of years already. It also came in spite of the fact that almost all our food was organically grown, most of it in our own garden and on our own farm.

As we learned more about candida, including the strange effects it can have on the emotions as well as on the physical aspects of the individual, we began to shift the blame for many of my chronic weird symptoms away from the hypoglycemia, which we had been blaming from 1975 onward, and toward candida overgrowth. We made this shift in 1987.

Knowing what we do now, we suspect that actually the yeast overgrowth and the blood sugar problems both contributed their share to the strange sensations I was experiencing both physically and mentally. So did the direct effects of chemicals in the environment. But I'm getting ahead of my story again; I'd had lots of chemical exposures previous to 1987, but not until that year did we learn what they can do to the body and the mind of susceptible individuals.

Each of the imbalances discussed above makes the other worse. With the little knowledge we had at the time, combined with the fact that our doctor knew nothing at all about these maladies, is it any wonder we were at a loss to know just where to turn for help?

Nystatin and its Effects for Me

I mentioned in the first section of this chapter that in the fall of 1987 I found a non-orthodox medical doctor who was willing to treat my candida with nystatin. He told me up front that with my degree of candida overgrowth, it would take at least two years for the nystatin to do its job.

Within a few weeks on the drug, however, each dose was making me so nauseated that I decided I'd rather live with the candida than with the constant urge to throw up. The nausea lasted twenty-four hours a day.

The three months I took nystatin didn't bring any noticeable relief from the candida. They did, however, bring a worsening of my chemical symptoms—something that isn't supposed to happen once you're on nystatin. Now, the least trace of smoke in the air would stop my breathing. Synthetic fabrics against my skin would cause a more instant reaction than ever before, driving me almost out of my mind with itching. I also began to react to several foods—something I had never done before. Potatoes would leave me feeling like a wet rag. I also began to react much more dramatically to mold than I ever had before.

When the nystatin failed me, I came almost to the threshold of despair. All I really wanted was release, and I often asked the Lord to take me Home.

New Diagnosis: Chronic Fatigue Syndrome

The doctor who prescribed the nystatin for me said that I had chronic fatigue syndrome—a relatively new diagnosis at the time. By this time, we had somewhere picked up the fact that fibromyalgia (chronic, constant muscle aching over the entire body) is associated with chronic fatigue syndrome. Earlier, I had accepted the verdict of the doctor who cared for me when I had the rheumatic fever: the total body aching would stay with me for the rest of my life.

With a diagnosis of chronic fatigue syndrome now, my symptom picture began to make at least a little sense. The doctor who gave the nystatin said that once the candida came under control, the fibromyalgia would lessen as well. So would many of my other symptoms.

Unfortunately, his only weapon was nystatin. When it failed me, he had nothing more to offer. Oh, well, at least he acknowledged that my problems had real physical causes. That was more than most of our friends would do.

An Alternative Approach

About the time I quit the nystatin, I found Dr. Theron Randolph's book Alternative Approach to Allergies at the public library. By this time I was struggling with many problems. Hypoglycemia. Candida yeast overgrowth. Chronic fatigue syndrome. Glandular imbalances. Female problems, notably severe PMS. Chemical sensitivity. Overweight. Chronic bronchitis. Constant constipation.

My constellation of symptoms overlapped and intermeshed, reinforcing each other in such a way that they constituted not one but half a dozen interlocking, pernicious circles.

We read Dr. Randolph's book early in 1988. It made us wonder whether my current problems—the chronic pain, the terrible tiredness, the chemical sensitivity, and the inability to think—might all be mature manifestations of my various childhood illnesses. I had gone from growing pains to fibromyalgia; from bronchitis to tonsillitis and constant colds; from acne to rough, dry legs and callused, cracking heels; from cold sores and constant sties to frequent canker sores; from asthma to overbearing tiredness; from joint stiffness to outright arthritis; from absent-mindedness to a cotton candy brain. Might there be some connection between all these problems and my present overriding sensitivity to chemicals in the air I breathed?

Had we been mistaken all along in thinking of each as a separate entity? Had we taken a piecemeal approach to the integral parts of one great continuum? Did my whole health history constitute a cascade of seemingly unrelated problems for which the cause or causes were the same? Could one set of predisposing conditions have laid the foundation for all these imbalances? Set the stage for such a variety of symptoms?

The more we studied Dr. Randolph's work, the more we believed that the above was the case. Also, the more convinced we became that the unending parade of mental and emotional symptoms I had experienced for many years and was still experiencing found its roots in the same physical imbalances as were allowing the continuing development of various physical manifestations. Both hinged upon my sensitivity to chemicals in the air.

Why were my Responses Inconsistent?

The inconsistency of my responses to chemicals had puzzled me for years. This failure of my system to respond the same way to the same irritant from one exposure to another posed a tremendous hurdle both for me and for the people around me. If I was really so ill, then why didn't my responses follow some consistent, predictable pattern? Why did an exposure I could tolerate well one day make me desperately ill the next? And the day after that then, the same irritant might not cause any response at all.

At this point in the story—early 1988—I was still at the stage where the only predictable thing about my response to chemicals was that my response would be unpredictable. (After the sensitivity snowballed late in 1989, that changed: I then reacted both regularly and dramatically to every chemical irritant I encountered. But for the first fourteen years that I had the problem, my responses were consistently inconsistent.)

The Concept of Total Load

I don't remember at what point I first read Dr. Sherry Rogers' book, The E I Syndrome. (E I stands for Environmental Illness.) There I learned the concept of total load. This concept clarifies why the mildly to moderately sensitive person might react in different ways at different times to the same irritant.

The degree of response, Dr. Rogers explains, depends upon the total load the person's system has accumulated and is carrying at the moment of exposure to a given irritant.

Many factors modulate the person's response. Is he well rested or tired? How intense is the concentration of the chemicals to which he is exposed? How much time has elapsed since he last encountered a similar irritant? Has he been eating wisely or foolishly during the past few days? Is his elimination up to par? Does he have a cold or some other infection? Is he under pressure in some other way—a deadline to meet, for example?

These factors as well as many other variables can make a difference in the susceptible person's total load. That difference in his total load then alters his body's responses to whatever irritant he might be facing at the moment. And the response of the body dictates the reaction of the brain. If the body is able to handle the exposure, molecules of the irritant don't get into the brain tissue. If they do get in, they can cause a host of seemingly mental symptoms. These mental symptoms are then taken as proof that the person has either a spiritual or an emotional problem, and needs counseling.

The person who is living in a setting where he is routinely exposed to low levels of chemicals in the air—levels that don't cut off his breathing, give him a headache, or make his eyes water—may still suffer from these mental effects of chemical exposure. But no one ever suspects that there's a physical basis for his problems.

Chapter Six

Housing That's Ecologically Sane

We had now read both Dr. Sherry Rogers' The E I Syndrome and Dr. Theron Randolph's An Alternative Approach to Allergies. By combining ideas from the two books, we concluded that an ecologically sane house—a relatively chemical free structure—would provide an environment that would relieve my battered immune system of the constant stress of chemical overload. This, according to the theory, should give my body an opportunity to heal. Once healing had taken place, I should be able to function normally again—or so we thought.

We designed and contracted the house ourselves, and it was built in the summer of 1988. The designing process was difficult for me, for my mental powers had already deteriorated considerably by this time.

There might be some value in reviewing here our housing arrangements over the dozen or so years preceding the building of the ecologically sane dwelling. In the summer of 1975, we renovated the old house we were then living in. Very soon after that, I began to have my first reactions to such things as diesel fumes and insecticides. Then in 1977, we built and moved into the superinsulated house. That, of course, was followed by many bizarre symptoms, which at the time we didn't realize had any connection to the chemicals exuded by all those new building materials.

In 1981, we sold the superinsulated house and moved to an area where the summers didn't last so long and weren't so hot. There, we lived in an old farm house that hadn't had renovations for many years. I was reasonably well for a couple of years, until once again we undertook renovations. At this point, impossible as it might seem, we had still not established any connection between how I felt and the house I lived in.

Soon after the renovations (including building an entire new wing) were completed, I was once again suffering from really weird symptoms. But not until we read the books mentioned above and then talked to the naturopathic doctor did we understand what might be happening.

Soon after we moved into the ecologically sane house, we thought we were beginning to see some improvements. The changes we saw came slowly, however, and were so small that we soon began to wonder whether I didn't imagine them.

We soon decided that overall the house hadn't made any significant difference in my sensitivities. At this point, we didn't yet realize that just the fact that I was no longer getting worse was at least some progress in the right direction.

So the house failed to provide the kind of help I had hoped for. Later, we realized that Dr. Randolph wasn't promising recovery from the allergic reactions by living in a relatively chemical-free setting. His emphasis focused mostly on enhancing the ability to cope with life by removing oneself from the stressors. It was my idea that by avoiding chemicals for a certain period of time I would gain resistance to them. Dr. Randolph had promised no such thing.

Later on, we did learn that in the earliest stages of sensitivity, avoidance of chemicals is sometimes enough to bring about recovery. Once the body is freed from its load of allergens, it can regenerate its resistance. This then allows it to detoxify further chemicals as they come in.

When Nothing is Left but Avoidance

When the new house failed to give me the help I'd hoped it would, I finally decided that all that was left was avoidance. But being a person who thoroughly enjoys other people, I found that decision difficult to make. For in order to avoid chemicals in the air, I also had to avoid people.

So in spite of knowing that each exposure lowered my resistance to chemicals even further, I continued to circulate in society to a limited extent. However, I now functioned on the fringes of the crowd, always keeping to places that offered access to fresh air the moment I could no longer breathe.

We did totally maintain the chemical-free environment at home. No chemical substances came into our house except unscented laundry powder. (I've since learned that a mixture of half Borax and half washing soda makes a perfect substitute for laundry powder, and has no scent at all. Clothing washed in this mixture will smell fresh and clean, at least if it's dried out of doors. I don't know how well it would work to take out grease; we don't have mechanics in our family.)

During this phase of my illness, I became an expert at holding my breath. Whenever I got close to something I couldn't tolerate, I'd see if I could wait it out, holding my breath until the offending substance moved on its way. Or, if the substance was on a stationary object, holding my breath until I was out of its way.

One Food a Day Experiment

We'd been living in the ecologically sane house for almost a year when I embarked upon another experiment. I had read that sometimes people with chemical sensitivity are allergic to some food or foods they eat every day. This allergy makes their sensitivity to chemicals worse, because the presence in the body of allergenic foods weakens the immune system.

I therefore went onto a diet of just one food per day—bananas, for instance, or boiled brown rice, or eggs. Things such as bread, which are actually a combination of various food items, were avoided altogether. So were all the foods that

I normally ate more often than once a week.

The information I had read said to eat this way for several weeks; then gradually reintroduce the foods that had previously been eaten frequently. Any negative response upon again eating a given food would indicate an allergy that I hadn't previously been aware of.

This diet had a major unforeseen effect: I totally lost my appetite. After just a few days on it, I had to force myself to eat at all. I simply wasn't hungry. Because I'd been very much overweight for years, we were delighted to see the pounds roll off. I lost twenty-eight pounds in forty-two days. I'd never been able to lose like that before.

Repercussions from the Sudden Weight Loss

So far as the original intention of the one-food-a-day diet was concerned, we felt that it failed miserably: I became more sensitive to chemicals in the air than I'd ever been before. This made no sense whatsoever to us. Losing weight is supposed to make a person feel better. Why, then, did it make me so much more sensitive?

I had lost about twenty pounds when my sensitivity to chemicals took a sudden, dramatic turn for the worse. Never had I experienced anything like this before. At first we thought I had just caught up to the point where I would have been anyhow had we never built the ecologically sane house. But soon I had gone far beyond the point that I would have been at had we not made that change.

Later on we learned a logical explanation for what had happened. But at the time we were totally perplexed. It seemed that no matter what we did in an effort to help my difficulties, either it didn't help or else it made matters worse.

As stated above, I stayed with the one-food-a-day diet for a full six weeks. During that time my level of sensitivity increased to the point that even the residual dry-cleaning fluid, fabric softener, or scented laundry powder in people's clothing left me muddle-brained and light-headed and unable to get my breath. No one dared to visit me unless he made himself as fragrance-free as possible, including airing his clothing outdoors for several hours ahead of time.

I don't blame the people who couldn't go to all that bother. Looking back, it's easy enough to understand why our friends decided I was likely insane. What would I have thought of someone who had the same symptoms as I did, if my affliction had fallen on them instead of on me?

As it was, my husband and I and our children found ourselves floundering severely in our own efforts to grasp what had happened. Along with our friends, we had already had difficulty accepting the reality of my earlier sensitivity levels. It's not much wonder that the sort of reactions I was describing now left both them and us dumbfounded. None of us had ever heard of anything like this before.

No Hope...No Hope

The medical interview detailed in the first chapter of this book took place at this time. Now our doctors deserted us too. It was one more reason for me to feel alone. I began to visualize myself as hopeless—a jellyfish afloat on an ocean in which the currents had no mercy, and where the insidious undertow would someday swallow me whole.

Although I hadn't completely given up on life earlier, I now felt that there was no more reason to hope. I was helpless against an array of physical and emotional and mental imbalances that I somehow knew had the power to destroy me. The unwilling victim of a haphazard complex of weird, almost eerie aberrations that tormented me without warning one after another and often simultaneously, and over which I had not the least control.

Is It a Spiritual Problem?

People who are covering up something they know is wrong will sometimes manifest physical, emotional, or mental symptoms (or a combination of any of the three) as a direct result of having hidden sin in their lives.

Some of these symptoms might appear to be purely physical, such as chest pains or indigestion. Others might present as emotional factors, such as defensiveness or hostility. Still others might seem to be totally mental, such as memory loss or the inability to think clearly and come to logical conclusions.

There is no question that hidden sin can and in some cases does lead to such disorders. The stress of knowing that he's hiding something he should repent of, reveal, confess wherever appropriate, and forsake, can cause a person to manifest some very strange behavior.

On the other hand, it is also true that physical imbalances in the body, particularly those imbalances that affect the brain tissue, can lead to some very strange symptoms and behaviors. This is because the brain is physical tissue; when you die, your brain will decay just as the rest of your body will.

This physical brain tissue is responsible for processing your thoughts. If it is physically compromised, the thinking might become distorted. Distorted thinking, in turn, can lead to distorted behavior.

Given the above, it seems logical to conclude that the person whose behavior is distorted might or might not be covering up some sin in his life. He also might or might not be experiencing some purely physical imbalances that are leading to his strange symptoms. His responses might be generated by a combination of both spiritual and physical irregularities. (The man who's hiding sin might also have blocked coronary arteries that cause him to experience chest tightness or pain.)

To conclude that all problems that manifest as emotional or mental must be caused by only physical imbalances is just as illogical as it is to conclude that such problems must always indicate some spiritual irregularity. It would be rather shortsighted to decide that since drunk drivers go in the ditch sometimes, then all drivers who go in the ditch must be drunk.

From the moment I began to manifest strange symptoms as a result of exposure to chemicals in the air, there were those who concluded that I had serious spiritual problems. Well-meaning and sincere brethren were convinced my symptoms indicated that I must be hiding some sin in my life. They kept encouraging me to confess it, assuring me that once I had done so all would be well.

Some people, under such pressure, do make confessions—sometimes myriads of them. Sometimes they confess to things they never even thought of doing. They're as desperate for answers as anyone is—maybe more so. After all, they're the ones who have to live with the strange manifestations of the problem.

My nature was such that I wasn't given to inventing confessions, even if others wanted me to make them. The symptoms of my illness were very real, and I could see no value in pretending otherwise. I knew that pretending my headaches and inability to breathe were caused by some hidden sin that wasn't there couldn't help.

As I said above, those who thought I must be hiding sin were as sincere as they could be. They were trying hard to help me; I understand that better now than I did at the time.

To help understand their position, we must remember that I experienced sensitivity to chemicals long before it was common. I was the first person either we or our friends had ever heard of who couldn't breathe in the presence of strong perfume. It isn't hard to understand, looking back, that when such physical manifestations of my sensitivity were combined with the mental and emotional aspects involved, those around me would conclude that I had spiritual problems.

Moreover, the medical doctors had no answers. (They still don't.) We finally accepted that fact. Our friends, on the other hand, continued to feel that if I was really physically ill, then medicine must have an answer for me. Since it didn't, then my problems must be either psychological or spiritual in nature.

A few years earlier, I would have arrived at a similar conclusion about anyone who claimed to have my plethora of seemingly unrelated symptoms. I understand why others thought as they did.

But was the root of the problem actually spiritual? Did some spiritual renewal precede my recovery? If so, I am unaware of it—and I do think that I would have known it if I had somewhere along the way confessed whatever it was I had been (supposedly) hiding.

We do know that a great deal of physical adjustments were made in my diet and lifestyle in the months before I began to get well. We also know that I began to use a truly amazing amount of food supplements at the nutritionist's direction. For quite some time, I swallowed well over a hundred assorted pills, plus several powders and liquids, every day. (Please note that I'm ahead of my story here; the nutritionist hasn't come yet. I'm telling you about it here, however, because it fits into the subject we're discussing at the moment.)

So if you experience problems that you think are being generated by chemicals, and those around you think of them as evidence of spiritual irregularities, please give due consideration to their concerns. Search your own heart, and ask the Lord to search it for you, to determine whether there might be a basis for their suspicions. After all, it won't help to buy and swallow supplements, change your diet, or make other lifestyle changes if the problem is caused by hidden sin.

If in fact your problems are physical, don't do as I did, allowing yourself to harbor resentment against those who misunderstand you. They are doing their best; relate to them accordingly. Even when people thought that my problems were the figment of my imagination, I had no excuse to harbor the frustration and resentment did. I understand that now.

God is still in control, and nothing that comes your way has escaped His notice. I've experienced spiritual growth as a result of my illness that I might well have missed had I always been well. I needed the things He allowed to come my way.

Chemical Snowballing

Snowballing, when used in relation to sensitivity to chemicals, refers to a sudden, intense increase in a person's level of susceptibility. During a period of only a few weeks, a person might change from being moderately affected by chemicals in the air to experiencing truly serious reactions to them. At the same time, the amount of any chemical that can be tolerated becomes much less. Moreover, many substances that hadn't previously made any problem begin to cause reactions, some of them extreme.

I was already snowballing at the time of the interview with my doctor that I told about at the beginning of chapter one. My level of sensitivity had grown almost unbelievably during the preceding eight weeks. This sudden recent increase in my symptoms helped me to accept the doctor's verdict; I was now so sick that I didn't want to live.

Until all these things happened to me, I would have been the first to suspect that anyone who claimed to have symptoms such as I now had must be out of his mind. It's no wonder to me that by the time of that final doctor visit, only my family believed in me at all any more, and although they didn't say so in my presence, I'm sure they often wondered too whether Mother was insane.

During the very worst of my chemical troubles, we did find comfort in the fact that there were other people who had symptoms similar to mine. We didn't know any of them, but from reading we did know they were out there somewhere.

About six months after the snowballing finally let up, we came upon some actual statistics. Approximately 10,000 people in North America were then suffering from susceptibility to chemicals that was severe enough to confine them to their homes. (I was one of the 10,000, of course.)

Our first reaction to these figures was, that's a lot of people. But then we did some calculations, and discovered that 10,000 North Americans is about one person for every 35,000 of the population. When we realized that, we were better able to understand why neither we nor our friends knew anyone else who had an illness like mine. Was it any wonder that very few believed me?

The snowballing propelled me through more levels of sensitivity in four months than I had experienced in the previous fifteen years. Like a runaway train on a downhill track, I couldn't find a convenient place to stop. No one understood what had happened to me, least of all we who were closely involved. No one knew how to relate to me and my bizarre illness. I might as well have had bubonic plague.

Unclean ! Unclean !

We learned of the above statistics some time in 1990. At least we knew then that others—many others, in fact—were suffering the same sort of problems as I was. That afforded some comfort.

But as our doctor had told me during that final interview, I had gotten into this chemical sensitivity business somewhere near the leading edge of its development. My responses, therefore, were always ahead of anything the people around us were aware of. Thus, by the time my reactions had gotten exquisitely tuned, it wasn't exactly unusual for people to know that certain individuals were now experiencing the kind of responses that I had lived with fifteen years earlier.

But asking anyone to believe the stories I told about my present condition was just too much. We understand; it was too much for us too. Given the strangeness of my malady (I really did look like—and probably was at times—a mental case), it's no wonder no one was in the market for our opinion.

Given the amount of information available to them at the time, others' unbelief was justified. That didn't make either the illness or our friends' refusal to believe in it any less devastating to me at the time, however.

The snowballing left me as a social outcast . Not only could I not cope with people because of the fragrances they carried with them, but they couldn't cope with me because they thought I was out of my mind.

I felt like a twentieth-century equivalent to the Old Testament lepers, with their agonizing separation from their fellows and their spirit-rending cry "Unclean ! Unclean !"

Chapter Seven

Why Did My Sensitivities Snowball?

We didn't know the answer to this question until several months further into the story. But for the sake of making sense to you, I've chosen to explain the reason here. (It was the nutritionist who told us what had happened.)

We had been tremendously pleased with my weight loss on the one-food-a-day diet. Unknown to us, however, the sudden loss was creating further problems for me that we were totally unaware of at the time. We had no idea that my body was storing huge amounts of toxins in its tissues. (When, under the nutritionist's guidance, I later began to dump this accumulated garbage, we truly were astounded at the nature and amount of it that came out of my body.)

When I lost all that weight so suddenly, the toxins were concentrated into a smaller body than they had been before. Therefore, the amount of toxin per pound of body weight became greater than it had been. This greater concentration of toxins renders the compromised body even less able to detoxify new supplies of chemicals as they gain access to the tissues—and that is at least a part of the reason why I became so much more sensitive to them at this time. (A much simplified explanation, but at least it helps.)

When we finally learned about the contribution body toxicity makes to chemical sensitivity, we wondered why none of the reading we had done had ever mentioned it. Later, we did find some such references. But at the time we needed this information most, we simply didn't have it.

We know, however, that the Lord allowed it to happen that way, and therefore it must have been for our good in ways that we did not yet understand.

A Look at the Snowballing Process

Both the intensity and the scope of my sensitivities to chemicals had been gathering momentum for a dozen years before the snowballing got under way. But when the snowballing began very early in the fall of 1989, we quickly came to realize that this was something entirely different from anything I'd ever known before. By the middle of that November, my reactions to chemical fumes in the air had reached levels I had never dreamed possible—and we still had no inkling why the level of sensitivity had suddenly gone berserk.

Six months earlier, I had to give a wide berth to anyone with fresh perfume. Now, a trace of fragrance that no one else could even detect left me nauseated and fighting to maintain consciousness as well as unable to breathe. My symptoms increased so severely and so quickly that by the end of the year I found it difficult to grasp, let alone to accept, the degree to which they had mushroomed.

Why did the sensitivity snowball like that? Maybe we'll never know. It could have just been the next step in the disease process. But we're inclined to agree with the nutritionist's view, as stated in the first section of this chapter. The weight loss had allowed a degree of concentration of toxins per pound of my body weight that was simply more than my system could tolerate as it was, let alone adding more.

We now know that had I gone through several months of

colon cleansing first, thus unloading some of the poisons from my tissues, the sudden weight loss probably wouldn't have led to the snowballing process. A cleaner body—and especially a cleaner liver—would have been able to handle the extra demands put upon it by the sudden loss of weight.

How Sensitive Can One Get?

Our family had absolutely no concept of how extreme chemical sensitivity can become. Many strange new things happened to me during the snowballing months, and I personally questioned my sanity many times.

Some time before the snowballing began, my family had taken to playing bloodhound. They would sniff out the places I wanted to go before I entered them. If they couldn't detect anything they knew would bother me, I would be able to tolerate the setting. Now, however, the sniff test sometimes failed. They would check as carefully as usual, and think that all was well. But the moment I would enter the room, I'd be in trouble with my breathing. We all found that hard to accept. It had worked before; why should it not work now?

At about this same time I started to taste the presence of chemicals when they were at levels too low for even my nose to detect. I'd experience a burning, metallic sensation behind the tip of my tongue. I soon learned that when I sensed this offensive essence of chemicals it was time for me to get out of the area—even if I couldn't smell a thing.

This stretched our friends' ability to believe beyond its limits. It did ours too. And yet, whether we liked it or not, I was now saying, "Something in this room makes me ill!" when no one, myself included, could smell a thing.

Every time I became sensitive to a substance that hadn't bothered me before, or even when old irritants brought forth more severe symptoms than they had earlier, we would allow ourselves to hope that now the reactions were as severe as they could get. After all, didn't I some day have to reach some sort of zenith—some ultimate level beyond which such reactions could not go?

But every time, we soon learned that further exposure had the power to create yet more exquisite sensitivities. The extreme degree of my reactions had reached the point where it dazzled our senses as much as it did anyone's. And still, it seemed, the end was not by and by.

This is Supersensitivity

By the time the snowballing was over, licking a postage stamp made me feel like a wet rag, too limp to sit up in a chair. This weakness would last for as much as half an hour. (It wasn't related to fish-based glue: I ate fish without a problem.)

We had bought a portable air purifier so that I could take it along to church and other places where people wore perfume. By sitting right beside it I could be there on the fringe of the crowd. But within a few weeks of getting it I became sensitive to the fumes from the electric motor that drew the air through the filters in the machine. From that point onward, I had an unbelievable susceptibility to the fumes from electric motors—a degree of sensitivity I found incredible.

This became so acute that if I wanted to run the blender in my kitchen I'd have to go to the door first and stock up on fresh air. Then I'd hold my breath to actually operate the machine. I'd also have to air out the kitchen after the blender had been used before I could breathe in there again.

Other things that had never created significant problems began to cause reactions for which I had no explanation. The slightest whiff of liquid paper (white out) made me feel as though I might pass out as well as cutting off my air supply.

The sensitivities became ever more exquisitely tuned, until an ordinary ball-point pen within a foot of my face made my eyes go out of focus and left me feeling nauseated and unable to breathe. When one's ability to cope in society is seriously compromised by a close encounter with a ball-point pen, it's understandable that people wonder what is going on.

Sometimes now, too, when others detected the presence of perfume, I wouldn't sense any fragrance at all, but I would experience an especially unpleasant smell—an acrid chemical odor—and would taste the horrible, burning, metallic sensation on my tongue.

I got to the point where upon occasion I'd neither smell nor taste anything out of the way at all; I would just be suddenly short of air and very, very ill. There seemed to be no explanation for these incidents, but moving into fresher air would always bring relief.

Was I a Universal Reactor Now?

The only definition I've ever seen of a universal reactor is "a person who responds negatively to almost everything all the time." By the end of November of 1989, I fit the description well. The few substances that didn't bother (mostly foods) were more than compensated for by the severity of my reactions to the things that did make me problems.

White potatoes and corn flakes made me faint and confused, and my body would feel as if my bones had turned to jelly; I might flow off my chair the way a strip of cooked spaghetti slips off a fork. Wheat made me feel extra well for a while, but the high would be followed by a headache that would last for several hours.

Pollen, dust, and animal dander, which had bothered me only slightly earlier, now became enough of a problem to make me avoid them. Mold, which had bothered me ever since my months on nystatin, became a serious irritant. I couldn't breathe if someone opened a jar of home-canned food that had developed mold on its surface. Going into a moldy building was out of the question.

But chemicals in any and every form were my particular nemesis. As explained above, even a trace that no one, myself included, could detect, closed my airways, made me nauseated, and gave me a headache. They also left me feeling desperately weak—a weakness that's impossible to describe.

Brain Fag

During the downhill slide in the fall of 1989, the mental fogginess called brain fag also snowballed. My powers of comprehension deteriorated astonishingly. The misunderstandings of my friends were hard enough to endure. The social restrictions were difficult indeed for me to accept. But worse yet was the constant deterioration of my memory and the loss of the capacity to reason. Increasingly, I complained, "I just can't think!"

Nor could I remember anything. Reading, which I had always enjoyed, became an exercise in futility. From line to line, I couldn't remember the story. I couldn't remember what I read in the Bible either, but the Scriptures left me with comfort and peace, and with none of the frustration brought by any other reading material I tried.

I knew the meanings of the words in a story. It was the plot that threw me. Even stories designed for little children left my brain in a whirl: from one paragraph to another, I'd lose the writer's train of thought.

I could learn nothing new, and most of the things I had known earlier had sunk beyond retrieval, suffocating in the mental quagmire that occupied the space once housing a relatively normal brain.

Cotton Candy Brain

Short-term memory became a cruel joke. Within ten seconds the simplest message had sunk beyond the point of possible recall. To dial a telephone number, I had to check the phone book digit by digit, and I'd cover each one as I dialed it, for otherwise I couldn't remember how much of the number I'd already dialed. A few years earlier, I could zip through long-distance calls, area code included, after looking at the complete number just once.

But now so many things were out of joint. Like a blindfolded man on a roller coaster, I had no point of reference to pin anything down. Writing reminder notes to myself didn't help; I'd find them lying about the house, indisputably in my handwriting, but outdated and beyond recall.

In the midst of such mental chaos, I still had about two days a month when I could actually think. But most of the time my brain functioned like a ball of cotton candy, minus only the color and the taste. A numb, gray, swirling emptiness—a kaleidoscope that had lost its colored glass.

Why should death not offer sweet release? Blissful deliverance from the physical pain that had gone to bed with me every night and risen with me every morning for three-quarters of my life? Freedom from the outright unbelief most of the people around me expressed concerning my sensitivities? Escape from the numbing inertia that seemed to be coiling ever more suffocatingly around my brain?

I was waiting in a hurry now to leave this world behind. Death wore the face of my greatest ally, and heaven offered incalculable gain. Where could I possibly want to go but Home?

Chapter Eight

Panic!

Before I ceased to snowball, I encountered another monster: blind, unreasoning, uncontrollable fear. The least hint of something that might make me ill would send a cascade of panic through me. Was this because I dreaded to face yet another situation where I'd not be able to breathe? I was certainly tired of being made a spectacle of by my need to dash off to get clean air.

Or might the panic have resulted from a direct influence of the chemical irritant on the tissues of my brain? Some allergens can cross the blood-brain barrier, thus making direct contact with the tissues of the brain. Authorities on the subject say that when this happens, the irritants have the power to alter the biochemical functions that produce the mental patterns known as thought.

Our friends didn't understand that; they insisted that I could control the panic if I wanted to. If I couldn't, then I had a spiritual problem. They didn't realize, of course, that like the beating of the heart or the blinking of the eyes, the sort of reactions I was experiencing were beyond the control of the conscious mind. They are regulated by the autonomic nervous system, which operates apart from the control of consciousness.

Our doctors knew these things, but they didn't have a clue what to do about them. As noted in the first part of chapter one, their only real conclusion was "go home and die."

Social Leper

As the snowballing progressed, I became too sensitive to the personal care products people use to be a part of any group unless I could sit right beside an open window or door. Even there, the air had to be coming in or I couldn't get my breath. If it was going out, it carried the aura of the people in the room; I couldn't breathe.

The weather was getting colder as the snowballing progressed, and it was often impractical to have a window open. Also, our church auditorium had windows only on the side where the men sat (we have separate seating for men and women.) So even on those days when the weather was mild enough to have windows open, there wasn't anywhere in that room that I could breathe. I missed being able to attend church services more than I minded anything else that this strange illness had brought my way.

The restrictions on my social life went far beyond church, of course. Stores, the bank, and the post office left me feeling as though I were strangling. Busy highways, with their diesel and other fumes were out of bounds. So were service garages and dry-cleaning shops. Drug stores and shopping malls left me dizzy and confused, and I'd not be able to breathe. Even the public library made me ill.

Nor is the above list complete. Anywhere that chemicals outgassed into the air, I couldn't go. That even included other people's houses; a bar of scented soap on the bathroom counter was enough to keep me out of the dwelling.

My life-long claustrophobia got worse as the number of things that made me unable to breathe increased. I became more and more cautious of situations where I might not be able to escape to clean air should my breathing reflex go on strike. As I snowballed, the concentration of offending molecules that was needed to stop my breathing continued to grow less. As a result, I became more and more conscious of the possibility that some day I might encounter a situation where I couldn't escape.

Several doctors had already suggested that I ought to carry oxygen with me at all times, just for such an event. (They knew my sensitivities were real.) I never did; I would rather have died than be caught using oxygen by someone who didn't believe I really had a physical problem. Was this just one more strange perversion in my thinking; the conclusion of a chemically intoxicated brain?

The clinical ecologist (allergist who specializes in sensitivity to things in the environment) with whom our family doctor had conferred had advised me to avoid the things that made me sick. That input would have been helpful for someone to whom the chemical problem was new, I suppose. But it didn't help me; I had already been avoiding a multitude of substances for quite a number of years. I had to avoid them just to stay alive.

More than I ever had before, I felt like a social leper.

Pernicious Inertia

I've been tired to one extent or another all my life. But now, along with the increase in my other complications, I experienced greater fatigue than I'd ever known before. This even surpassed the tiredness I'd felt following all the antibiotics I'd been given for pneumonia in the summer of 1978, which by now was eleven years in the past. An overpowering weariness now controlled greater and greater portions of my life. I spent fourteen hours of each twenty-four asleep.

During the hours I was up, I was weak and tired, having neither the initiative to plan things nor the strength to follow through on a project that I might, in a brighter moment, have begun. Mostly I sat in my rocking chair (we had already thrown out our stuffed furniture because the smell of the foam rubber in it made me ill), thinking very little and doing even less.

By November of 1989, even the light exertion of embroidering for a few minutes left me physically exhausted, absolutely drained. A trip from my chair to the sink required so much effort that I would often ask my husband or our daughter to bring me a drink of water.

The Hair-Trigger Response Continues

From the moment my sensitivities began to snowball, it seemed that the more chemicals I exposed myself to, the more speedily my reactions to them grew. After a certain point, sensitization begat further sensitization without any logic, pattern, or reason. Hair-trigger responses developed, sharpened to a point that even I thought went beyond belief.

One day, for example, I got out of our vehicle after having sat there for about an hour while waiting for the appointed time to go into the building nearby. I had gone only a few steps toward the back door when I became aware of something impeding my breathing. Reflexly, I held my breath. I hurried on. I'd get more air as soon as I passed the corner of the building.

But when I rounded the corner and gasped for breath, only half a lungful went in before my breathing stopped completely. The source of my problem was standing outside the back door of the building—a woman who was wearing fresh perfume. I had no clue of her presence until a split second after my breathing stopped.

I was grateful for such experiences; they verified the reality of my sensitivities. Without these occasional situations where chemicals I never could have suspected were there made me acute problems, I might have gone completely out of my mind with wondering myself whether or not my symptoms were generated by my imagination.

We still didn't understand why I had developed such sensitivites when other people who lived in the same environment as I did were still quite normal. But such experiences as the above helped to prove that my sensitivities were real. An irritant that I had absolutely no inkling was there, outdoors and more than seventy-five feet away from me, around a corner and at cross current rather than straight upwind from where I was, had distressed my airways enough to cause me to reflexly hold my breath. (I hadn't smelled anything fragrant; all I was aware of was that there was something here I couldn't breathe.) What further evidence could I need that the sensitivities were real?

No Means of Escape

A friend who read this manuscript before it was printed made the comment at this point that the reader is "lost and weary, wondering about the outcome of all these things." She suggested that I should "concentrate on the things we did that had positive effects toward recovery, skipping all the erroneous thinking and the efforts that didn't bring results."

When we discussed it with her, however, she agreed that there's a place for the story as it stands. For our family, too, was lost and weary, wondering about the outcome of all these things. And as far as things that had positive effects toward recovery went, at that point, there weren't any. The medical world had deserted us, and we didn't know where else to turn. By this point, I was so ill that I was looking forward to the only possible release we knew of—death.

Is Immunity Possible?

I knew that each exposure made the next one worse. Some folks, however, didn't agree. "You pamper yourself," they suggested. "If you won't expose yourself to your allergens, how can you expect to build up immunity to them?"

"But each exposure makes me more vulnerable," I replied. "The body isn't programmed to produce antibodies to chemicals the way it does to viruses and germs. No one has antibodies to chemicals. It's just that most folks can detoxify them as they come into their systems. I can't. (At this point, all we knew about why not was that somehow my immune system had gone out of kilter. We did know that this was tied in with candida overgrowth, but nystatin had failed me, and we knew of no other treatment for the yeast.)

I might as well have conserved my energy as to try to explain these things. It took a long time for me to accept the fact, but I finally understood that people weren't in the market for my story. They "knew" that my problems were all based on spiritual irregularities in my life.

To give credit where it's due, a few really had begun to wonder whether there might be some actual physical basis for at least some of what was happening.

One friend even seemed to feel some sort of obligation to find answers to what he had begun to suspect was a bona fide problem. I'll probably never forget the expression on his face or the frustration in his voice the moment he said, "It doesn't matter what I suggest; you say you already tried it and it didn't work!"

Why Not Take Shots?

By that time, of course, we had tried a lot of things. Who wouldn't have? I had not, however, had injections in an attempt to desensitize my body to the allergens.

"Why don't you go to an allergist for shots?" We heard the same suggestion several times. Having read in The E I Syndrome of the poor long-term track record for such a procedure when used for chemical sensitivities in general and for multiple sensitivities in particular, I wasn't eager to try that route.

But folks kept intimating that they'd never accept my symptoms as incurable until we had tried allergy shots. "Lots of people get relief from their allergies with shots," they argued. "Why don't you try them at least?"

There was no use trying to explain the difference between allergy to natural things like pollen and house dust and allergy to synthetics and chemicals. So at last I asked my doctor to contact a clinical ecologist for me. I would have the shots in spite of the dangers I knew they posed, and get well or die while trying.

The response from the allergy specialist, recorded in the first segment of this book (a single scratch test could be enough to end my life) put the idea of injections to bed once and for all. No one ever mentioned them again.

Immunity by Exposure?

Some folks still insisted that exposure to my allergens could build up my natural immunity to them. They still wouldn't listen to the fact that the human body doesn't build up immunity to chemicals; it either detoxifies them as they come in or else it doesn't. "How did I expect to become immune," they asked, "when I refused to expose myself to the substances that made my problems?"

By the time this pressure came, the snowballing had pretty well stopped. But I had reached the point that any environment (other than outdoors in clean air) other than our own house gave an instant metallic, burning sensation on my tongue. If I stayed a while in an exposure that was mild enough that I could still breathe, I'd go home with a raging headache that would last for the remainder of that day and all of the day following. Also, my eyes would refuse to focus properly for a number of hours.

In spite of all that, I still had to contend with the idea that by protecting myself from the trigger substances I was preventing my system from developing a natural immunity to them. Some of our friends even wondered whether avoidance of the irritants encouraged the development of further sensitivities.

Under the circumstances, is it any wonder I finally decided to prove them wrong or die while I was trying?

Chapter Nine

Enough Is Enough

From reading I had done earlier, I knew that the idea of gaining immunity by exposure to my allergens was faulty. The human body was never designed to become immune to chemicals. Nevertheless, I had to dispose of the suggestion somehow. And I knew how our friends wanted that done.

So one morning I set out to prove to myself once and for all whether or not they might be right about the source of my symptoms. My husband went to town, and I impulsively decided to go along—a thing I hadn't done for many weeks.

The last several trips I had taken to town had convinced me that the outing wasn't worth what it cost me anymore. The misery I endured while in the places of business would have justified that conclusion on its own. But when that aspect of the trip was combined with the chemical hangover that followed, I had more than enough reason to stay at home while my family did the shopping.

My decision to go again that morning was based on my determination to settle the issue permanently, at least in my own mind: either chemicals did or they did not make problems for anything but my imagination.

We stopped at the drugstore first. The aura of chemicals gave me the sensation of floating in the air, but when I looked at my feet they were still on the floor. So I stuck it out, waiting for the pharmacist to fill our daughter's prescription.

From the drugstore, I went to the bank. The lines were long, so my husband said that if I was sure I would be all right he'd go and do a quick errand somewhere else. I was already far into a chemical reaction from the exposure in the drugstore, and didn't sense anything in the bank to make things worse. So I stood in line to wait my turn.

Without warning, I suddenly felt as though I was being strangled. (Strangled is the proper word here. There was no gasping for air: I couldn't get any.) Turning around, I discovered that a cigar smoker had joined the line several spaces behind me. (Smoking was still legal in public buildings at the time.)

I gritted my teeth. It was no time to give up now. After all, I'd come to town specifically to gain immunity by exposure. And so, determined to prove whatever it was I thought I was proving, I struggled to keep breathing in spite of the cigar smoke. No running away as I'd so often done in the past when in the presence of an irritant.

It takes more than sheer determination, however, even when it's backed by a generous portion of stupidity, to overcome the sort of resistance my body was mounting to that smoke. I staggered out of the building, grasping at the wall for support, and collapsed in a heap on the sidewalk.

I still had the strength to keep massaging the breathing reflexes on my breastbone, hoping that soon I'd breathe again. By this point I was fighting unconsciousness as well as struggling for air. Everything had begun to turn dark around me when the breathing reflex finally cut back in. With a tremendous effort, I drew in a partial lungful of cold but acceptable air.

My husband found me there on the sidewalk and helped me to our vehicle. When he was sure I was all right again, he went and did the banking. When he came back, he wondered if

I was ready now to admit defeat. But by this time, my mental processes had been altered by the chemicals and I was ready to go to a greater extent than ever before to prove to myself that I had been wrong all along or to die in the process of trying.

So I persisted in my ridiculous crusade. The grocery store. (Not the detergent aisle however; I hadn't been in one of those for years.) The chiropractor's office. Even the waiting room in the service garage. By this time I felt as though whatever brain tissue I had started the day with had evaporated and been replaced with a wad of cobwebs.

The final stop was at the newspaper office where we had to pick up some printed materials we had ordered earlier. By the time we had finished our business there, I was finished too, even though I had spent more time on the steps in front of the building than inside.

By the time we headed for home, I felt worse than I had ever felt in my life. My eyes were out of focus. I felt as though someone had tightened a vise around my chest, and every little while they gave the handle another turn. My airways hurt so badly that every breath was torture. I was nauseated and weak to the point of staggering. My brain felt as if someone had pulled the plug, shutting off the current. All that was left inside my skull was a rousing headache.

Looking back, I marvel at my own stupidity. I had experienced increasing levels of sensitivity to chemicals for twenty years already. What did I think I was doing anyhow?

At the time, however, I had focused my energies on proving, both to myself and to anyone else who might care to listen, that I had good reasons for avoiding the things that I insisted made me sick. My husband needed nothing proven to him. He had already gone through twenty years of these things with me, and he was convinced that I was desperately ill.

Five-Day Hangover

The chemical hangover from the massive exposure lasted for five days and nights. Not only did I feel absolutely rotten all over physically, but my brain went into a longer tailspin than it ever had before.

Five days later, I began to recover from the effects of my foolishness. At that point my eyes still wouldn't focus well enough for me to read. It didn't matter: I couldn't comprehend anything anyhow. This one massive exposure, followed by its hangover, had taken more away from me intellectually than I had ever guessed could have happened in so little time.

When, in the aftermath of the exposure, I felt as close to being normal again as I got, my sensitivities had peaked at a level they had never approached before. More than ever, I was desperate to die.

Was it worth it to have proved to myself that chemicals really did make me grossly ill? Hadn't I known that already? What, then, did I gain?

Perhaps one thing: our friends who saw me during the hangover at last believed. Some even acknowledged that it was possible that I was beyond the point of medical help. But no one had any answers, of course, least of all ourselves.

Is This the Zenith of Reactions?

With the level of sensitivity I had now reached, we wondered again if I'd attained to the zenith—the point beyond which the body could not go. Then I remembered having read somewhere that no matter how seriously you react to a given exposure today, you still have the potential to respond more dramatically tomorrow.

Well, as far as I was concerned, the snowballing had gone far enough to do for the remainder of my life. I'd had enough of the toxic headaches and the sick-all-over feelings—the rousing chemical hangovers for which I knew no fix.

From now on, I'd be a good girl and protect myself from the things that made me ill, just as I'd been doing all along. I didn't have long to live anyhow. Did it matter what people thought of me and my sensitivities? Whether they believed that my symptoms were real or whether they thought I made them up to get attention? After all, I was the one who did the suffering. Other people would just have to think what they pleased.

Chapter Ten

Might Nutrition Help?

By the time of the visit to town recounted in the preceding chapter, I had already resigned myself to an early death. Soon after that trip, a nutritionist came along and insisted that he could help me if I'd do everything he told me to.

He blew my entire universe wide apart: he offered me life when I didn't want to live. I was already waiting in a hurry for the Lord to take me Home. Why would anything a nutritionist had to offer interest me now?

My family saw it differently; they wanted me to live. "What have you got to lose?" they challenged when I expressed reluctance to listen to what the nutritionist had to say. "If his system doesn't work for you, it could hardly make anything worse. You've always wanted to learn about herbs and stuff like that. Here's your chance!"

They thought that I could learn? Had they forgotten that nothing new lodged for more than ten seconds in my cotton candy brain? Who did they think they were fooling: did I want to learn?

I thought they had to be teasing. It turned out that they

weren't. I couldn't understand what they were thinking. Had they refused to believe that I was done with life? I think so, yes. In spite of my repeatedly saying so, they could not convince themselves that I wanted to die. That nothing really mattered now but Heaven.

Decision Point

Until the nutritionist came along, I'd had no choice but death. By resigning myself to it, I had done nothing more than give in to the inevitable. The doctors had already said I had a maximum of two years to live.

But now a decision had been thrown at me, confusing what had earlier been a clear-cut issue. Death? Or life?

It was the hardest choice I ever faced. I was already disheartened, burdened by the physical pain, by the unfounded emotional stresses, by the mental lasstitude, and by our friends' almost universal refusal to accept my sensitivities. My interest in life had waned until it was far outweighed by my anticipation of being with the Lord.

To my way of thinking, death meant merciful release. Escape from the social restrictions and from the feeling of suffocation that every chemical exposure brought. Deliverance from the inescapable crawling sensations that left me feeling so much of the time as though a million maggots were wriggling on my skin. Respite from the terrible exhaustion—the pernicious inertia—and from the trancelike uselessness of a body and mind deprived of the strength to care. Freedom from the relentless procession of days when I could not think.

Why should I turn back now? Why exchange the promise of warm, welcoming death, with no more sorrow, no more tears, and no more pain, for the vagueness and uncertainties of life?

The nutritionist offered no rosy visions of the road to recovery. He insisted he could help me, but he couldn't tell to what extent my faculties would return. What if my body would recover, but my mind, like a stained-glass window where the sunshine never falls, were left in the mist and shadows of the limbo it now endured? Wouldn't that be even worse than death?

Superimposed on the mental quagmire in which I already floundered, his offer of life churned up a relentless ferment of frustration and succeeded in driving me closer to despair.

Confusion of Terms

The course the nutritionist outlined presented hurdles of its own that I felt went beyond my ability to endure. "Expect to get worse before you begin to improve," he warned me on the phone when I first talked to him. "When chemical problems are as advanced as yours, it happens every time."

Get worse before I got better? I'd never heard of such a thing. Shouldn't any decent treatment make you feel better? At any rate, it shouldn't make you worse!

He spoke of a reversal process too—a going backward through the whole series of ailments that I had experienced in my lifetime. But I'd had all those things already; I never wanted them again.

He talked about tissue poisoning and intercellular garbage, and of cleansing the various organs and glands—in fact the entire body—from the accumulated toxins of the years.

It was all new to me, and none of the things he mentioned made a shred of sense. And certainly it didn't sound like fun. I wished I could better understand the things he was trying to explain to me. But though he tried hard, he couldn't force much useful information through the gray canopy of fog that swirled inside my head.

"Many imbalances preceded your chemical problems," he went on. "When sensitivities are as acute as yours are, we have to go to the very root of these imbalances. It's a nasty procedure, but I know of no other way; I certainly would tell you if I did."

My silent response was,"Maybe so. But it doesn't make sense to me." Out loud, I said, "I see." But that was all.

"I'm sure you can be helped to a great extent," he concluded. "But it's a little like cleaning a neglected house: we have to stir up a lot of dirt—scrape off many layers of filth and grime—before anything seems to improve."

The prospect definitely lacked appeal. Sick enough already,

why should I want to get worse? Even if getting worse was a part of ultimately getting better? Wouldn't the cure be more unbearable than the disease?

"I'll think about it," I hedged at last. "If I *do* decide I'm interested, *I'll* get in touch with *you*." The way I accented the sentence, he knew better than to call me back. We left it there while I made up my mind.

A Personal Choice

My family knew that I had suffered for many years already. Now they tried to accept the fact that I was looking forward to death. Therefore they said little from this point on. Some even apologized for having encouraged me to try the nutritionist's ideas.

Had they actually been able to feel the frustration of the intellectual no man's land in which I wandered day after purposeless day, I'm sure they would have willingly let me die. Perhaps only those who have faced such a decision head-on themselves—faced it when beleagured by the inabilty to think—will ever know the turmoil I went through in the following days.

Going on as I had been meant an almost airtight guarantee of death. Escape. Freedom. Release. No more pain or suffering or misunderstandings. No more of the cotton-swathed, gray morass of a world where I existed but could not function.

My family encouraged me to mind the Lord. But I had sought the Father's leading all along. When the doctors sent me home to die, I thought I had found it at last. Now, however, I was again at a decision point, and the choice was up to me. Warm, welcoming death? Or vague, uncertain life?

As I sought the Lord's direction during the next few days, a new consideration began to emerge—an idea that under the circumstances was so preposterous as to seem impossible. Yet I couldn't shake it off. What if my service on earth wasn't finished yet? Well, I would certainly have to realign my thinking if that were the case.

Could the Lord's having allowed the circumstances that

caused me to resign to death have been a test? And now that death was accepted—yea, welcomed—he offered me life instead? But the idea of going on living was harder than giving in to death had been.

What if I still had to live with pain? What if none of my other problems really went away, but just got enough better that I'd stay alive? The nutritionist had said I'd get better, but never really well. Was I ready for that?

My first response was,"Absolutely not!" Further reflection reduced it to,"Not yet."

"Whatever, Lord"

That was when I really started to say, "Whatever, Lord. No matter what I want, even more I want Your will for me."

I still believe, almost seven years later, that heaven approved of my resignation to death. I learned so much by it. But now I had to further discern the Father's will—to choose between the certainties of death and the uncertainties of life.

As the days of indecision passed, my degree of sensitivity to chemicals continued to increase. Unless I changed course soon, there likely wouldn't be any decision to make.

At last, I cried out in complete resignation, "Whatever, Lord. But You'll have to show me. I can't decide for myself."

Then very shortly, I knew the Father's will. Laying my selfish hopes of heaven aside, I had to give the nutritionist a try. Once again, I found satisfaction in yielding to the Father's perfect plan.

Ready to Proceed

Once I had made that decision, peace returned. Not the passive peace of resignation, but the confident assurance, in spite of what looked like insurmountable hurdles, that God does all things well.

We called the nutritionist the following afternoon and told him he could come. I couldn't go to the city to him, of course. Five different doctors had told me that strong perfume could kill me. How could I have possibly coped with a city?

A Word About Nutritionists, Etc.

Some warning is in order before you go to seek someone to advise you. There's a tremendous variation in the techniques used by those who give nutritional advice. Some simply analyze the symptoms and then suggest appropriate treatment. Others, who subscribe to the Eastern religions and other such occult connections, are not safe spiritually even if their treatments work. (Neither are some medical doctors; they, too, get involved in the occult sometimes. I've personally had an MD advise me to utilize a combination of biofeedback, self-hypnosis, and transcendental meditation to control my allergies to chemicals. He even told me he controls his own asthma that way.)

So find an adviser who totally shuns the "yin-yang" sort of thing, and who has nothing to do with the so-called "four elements." Run as fast as you can away from the practitioner who uses pendulums, pyramids, little black boxes whose function he can't explain, Ouija boards, magnets, and suchlike.

While we haven't thoroughly researched all of these, we do know that they're usually tied to the occult. Why would we expose ourselves to that in order to ascertain whether or not they're safe? A competent nutritionist who studies your symptoms thoroughly and who has a good working knowledge of the human body and its systems has no need of such devices to help with his job. He makes his judgments on the basis of how your body does and/or does not function. He forms his conclusions from your symptoms and from the condition of your body as well as from medical testing you may have had done.

On the other hand, he might ask questions that you can't see bear any relation to your problem. Be patient with him there so long as they're straightforward questions. He probably has a sound physiological reason for the things he wants to know. The body is an integrated unit, and the function of one part may be affecting another that's remote from it.

For example, often people with weak adrenal glands will cope very poorly with stress. So if he asks whether you go to pieces after an emergency is over, don't suspect his motives in wanting to know.

Chapter Eleven

We Meet the Nutritionist

A few days after we called him, the nutritionist came to our home. Knowing I'd need a great deal of information as well as encouragement, he arranged to stay long enough to get it all done. When he analyzed me, the first thing he found fault with was my liver.

I didn't tell you anywhere that three years before the nutritionist first came, I had been diagnosed by the medical world with two kinds of reproductive tract cancer. The more serious one disappeared during the anointing with oil service performed, according to the fifth chapter of the book of James in the Bible, by the elders of our church. However, the more common type was still there.

At that point we consulted a naturopathic doctor, and he, like the present nutritionist, found fault with my liver. "It's on strike," he explained. "And unless it comes back into line pretty soon, you don't have long to live."

He gave me supplements to take for it, of course. I took them faithfully, including several reorders, and assumed that all was well: the cancer disappeared. Retesting had shown me to be completely clear. Since the naturopath charged almost two hundred dollars an hour, we didn't go back to him. If we had, we might have learned that in the long run his liver treatment hadn't worked.

Now the nutritionist was complaining about my liver too. "It's sluggish," he explained. "Congested. Plugged full of poisons."

"So I'd better take something for it," I suggested.

He shook his head. "If you started at this point to take the things I give for liver, within three weeks you'd hate me so badly that you'd never consent to see my face again!"

"I see." I was puzzled. "So if my liver's in such a bad condition, why not go ahead and fix it?"

"Because it would make you awful sick, that's why. We won't dare to touch your liver for at least three months. Maybe four. I already told you to cleanse the colon first."

"But the naturopath I went to for the cancer never mentioned my colon," I argued. "Why did he give me liver things right away?"

The nutritionist ignored my question. "The things he gave for your liver helped for the moment, but over the long haul, what did you get?" he asked. "This time, let's try it my way and see what happens."

"What about blood purifiers then?" I asked next. "I've read about them in the herb book I have. Chapparal and echinacea and red clover—that kind of thing. Where do they come in?"

The nutritionist jumped as if somebody had shot at him. "Blood purifiers?" he yelled. "Blood purifiers, did you say?" His voice dropped back an octave or two, but his eyes were still rolled up toward the ceiling. "Listen to me! You could kill yourself with blood purifiers! And I'm not saying that to scare you, lady; it's a fact!"

He stared me down at point-blank range for a long time before he went on. "Maybe someday you can take blood purifiers," he conceded at last. "But that won't be for a very long time yet. *Do you understand?*" He was still staring at me.

"I see," I said. "Well, sorry I asked."

"I'm not!" he shot back. "I'm doubly glad you inquired.

Otherwise, I'd never have known you had any idea they exist."

"Doubly glad?" I asked. "How so?"

He grinned now, more relaxed. "First, we want to keep you alive while we get you well. And secondly, the people around here aren't very well acquainted with the type of supplements I use. We wouldn't want to give the products a black eye by letting you kill yourself with them."

After that, I didn't ask any more questions.

Take One Step at a Time

The nutritionist, however, wasn't finished with me yet. "You have to get this through your head: at the moment, you're in tough shape. Some people—like about ninety percent of the population—can take blood purifiers right off and get by with it. But a body like yours, with so much stacked up against it, can handle only a certain amount of challenges at once. You have to take it one step at a time—and the colon is the place you have to start. I've never in my practice seen a body as toxic as yours is, so take my word for it and stick with cleansing the colon for the present time."

"So what about all those wonderful builders you just finished telling me about, then?" I inquired. "I suppose I won't be able to take them either. After all the nice things you said about them, that's sort of a letdown."

Knowing what I now do about the builder category of supplements, I understand the long, defeated sigh with which the nutritionist greeted that particular piece of wisdom.

"Builders," he said slowly and very distinctly, "are a horse of a different color altogether. We'll start you on several builders right away."

I absorbed that information for a few moments before I suggested, "Maybe it would be best if you'd just write out a list of all the things I'm supposed to take, and for the moment I'll not ask any more questions."

"That," he said enthusiastically, "is an excellent idea!"

So for the first while I was on his program, I took exactly the varieties of supplements he suggested. But I still had to figure out for myself how much of each to use and how quickly I could increase the quantities. I also had to work out a way around the mineral supplements he wanted me to take. (More about that later.)

The Nutritionist Evaluates My Case

The nutritionist called both my liver function and my bowel activity into question right away. He also spoke of defective thyroid and of adrenal failure. My digestion came under question, too: he said it had almost ceased to operate. He talked of an overloaded colon and of tremendous candida overgrowth. Then he went on to discuss extreme body toxicity and immune system disregulation.

He spoke of cleansing the body and of rebuilding it, doing both at once if I were to get well. Not all of these concepts were totally new: I'd taken vitamins and minerals for years already. But this business of body cleansing—of making the inside as clean as the outside—well, that was a thought I'd never heard of before.

The very idea of a "clean colon" seemed a paradox. The colon existed as a sewer, I thought. A channel through which to dispose of body waste. By what stretch of the imagination could a sewer be made "clean"?

Why Colon Cleansing?

When you study the subject through, cleansing the colon makes abundant sense. When everything in the body works the way it ought to, the colon carries off about forty percent of the waste, which is quite a high proportion of the total. A colon that isn't in decent condition might not feel up to hauling its share of the load.

If the colon doesn't haul its share, what happens? First, the other channels of elimination become overloaded while they pinch-hit for the colon. This can lead to kidney, lung, and/or skin problems. And secondly, not all of the body's toxins get eliminated. Some of them get backed up into the system and stored in less active tissues, waiting for the day when circumstances arise that allow them to harm you.

So it's vitally important to keep the colon working up to its potential. If you have intestinal candida overgrowth—and I most certainly did—then the colon carries an even heavier burden. Then it's more vital than ever that it gets assistance first, before you begin to detoxify other tissues—tissues whose toxic waste must ultimately pass through the colon for elimination.

Once the colon is in decent working order (and that includes getting the candida growth under control), then you can dare to start cleansing the other parts of the body, beginning with the liver. After it's working relatively well, you can begin to use blood purifiers. They stir up garbage out of the tissues and dump it into the liver for detoxification before it's sent to the colon for elimination. A compromised liver can't handle that extra load—it's still clogged up with garbage of it's own. Therefore, each step must be taken in the proper order.

How to Cleanse the Colon

Once we understood that my colon was all gummed up with garbage, we were eager to start getting it cleaned up. But we knew absolutely nothing about the process.

"We use psyllium husk powder," the nutritionist explained. "When combined with water, it swells up and acts like a broom, sweeping the colon walls clean as it passes through.

"We also use the entire psyllium seed, ground very fine. This material, even though finely ground, still has a sanding action, and it grinds away at the garbage that's built up on the inside of the colon walls. Any fecal material that's adhering to the inside of the colon is thus removed. Until that stuff's gone, the colon can never function up to its potential.

"Besides the psyllium products, we also use cascara sagrada," he went on. "This pushes the fiber through more rapidly than it would go otherwise, which is important too. And the Naturalax 2 mixture conditions the colon walls, nudging them gradually toward regaining the normal function they have lost."

He also told us it would be necessary to drink additional water to keep the psyllium mixture soft so that it could pass easily through the colon.

My head was spinning with trying to remember all the things he was saying, and I began to wonder how I'd ever get it all accomplished.

"I'll help you," my spouse encouraged. "Just listen carefully, and together we'll remember enough to start, at least."

In the years since the nutritionist first came, we've learned that a multitude of products on the market are specifically designed for colon cleansing. Basically, they all consist mostly of psyllium seed and/or husk. Some have other herbs added to help move the material through the colon. Most of these taste pretty awful. We prefer to take the laxative herbs in capsules, swallowing them along with the psyllium.

Some folks sincerely believe that a real colon cleanser gives you cramps to tie you in knots. But such suffering isn't at all necessary. You don't have to suffer to get results. But you do have to move large volumes of psyllium and water through the colon. The bottom line, after all, is not how much did it hurt? But how much did it help?

Beware of products that promise to cleanse your colon in seven or eleven or twenty-one or whatever number of days. Anything that can be marketed will be marketed, remember. The average North American adult needs at least a year of persistent effort to accomplish colon cleansing. If you're a little older, and especially if you've had chronic constipation for years, it will take longer still. (Remember that in primitive societies, the norm is three bowel movements per day—and they don't use laxatives.)

If you start experimenting with colon cleansing and don't have a competent advisor, go slowly. Also exercise caution if you're buying some product for the purpose from someone who's new in the business. He may want you to consume large amounts of his products right away so that he can make more sales. We know one lady who met someone like that, and after a few days, she had to go to a colon therapist to get the psyllium reamed out of her colon. Someone who didn't know enough to tell her to drink abundant water with the psyllium had advised her to take far too much at the start. She had colon problems for years over that deal.

So start with just a level teaspoonful a day of the psyllium, and work up gradually. Usually you can get up to at least two level tablespoonfuls a day over a period of a month or so. Then hold it at that level for a long time, taking it consistently. Some folks use that much both night and morning. As I note in another place in this book, for a long while I used four heaping tablespoons of it every day.

Why Had I Stored Those Toxins?

During that first visit, the nutritionist told us that my entire body was burdened with garbage.

"You're literally suffocating in a load of poisons that you aren't aware of," he informed us. He then went on to explain that my perplexing illness was the result of a combination of various imbalances in my body. One of those imbalances was the accumulated garbage that my body somehow didn't know how to discharge.

"We don't know exactly what causes it," he said, "but some people's bodies tend to accumulate junk. It infiltrates the entire system, including the vital organs and glands. Some of it has been there for many years."

"Most of it comes from two sources," he went on. "First, the incomplete digestion of cooked foods, especially meats and other proteins. And secondly, constipation—which is anything less than three bowel movements a day."

"What about food additives and so on?" I inquired.

He shook his head. "I wouldn't say that's not involved, but the main culprits are the indigestion and the constipation. There are also toxins in the air and the water, and they do get into our bodies as well, but again, that's not the major problem.

"You'll never be well until you reduce your burden of stored poisons, no matter what sources they come from," he concluded. "That garbage is hindering your body from functioning properly, just as sludge buildup hinders the proper functioning of a motor."

It's almost seven years now since he told me those things. In all the studying I've done since, I still haven't found anything that really settles the question of why some people's bodies accumulate more garbage than other people's do. I have discovered that in the individual whose thyroid gland isn't working well, this tendency seems to be accelerated. So is his tendency to have a poor digestive capacity.

When digestion is poor, then particles of undigested food can get into the blood stream because they reach the part of the intestine where absorption is supposed to take place in their undigested state. From there, they can be deposited into the tissues of the body.

Constipation is a major contributor to the process of building up toxins in the tissues. And we know that constipation is often found in company with poor thyroid gland function.

We were amazed to learn from the nutritionist that constipation means anything less than three bowel movements a day. With a forty-five year history of chronic constipation, and probably the same duration of inadequate thyroid performance, I suppose it wasn't any wonder my body was stashed full of garbage. The marvel is that it hadn't already killed me.

Getting Regulated

My long history of constipation automatically demanded that I learn to use herbal laxatives. The nutritionist recommended two different types. Cascara sagarada is laxative only in nature. Nature's Way's Naturalax 2, on the other hand, combines laxative effects with colon-wall conditioning. Both are needed to restore normal bowel function.

The nutritionist wouldn't make any suggestion as to how many of each to use each day. I kept asking, but all he'd say was "Enough to keep everything moving through in eighteen hours or less."

Finally around the third or fourth time I asked, he yelled, "All I can tell you is, if it takes twenty, then take twenty!"

"Twenty?" I gulped. "Are you serious?"

He grinned. "I'd start with two," he said. "One of each. Take them once a day, and see what happens. Work up from there as you see you need more. And whatever you do, don't let the colon get stopped up!"

So I started with two a day. Three weeks later, I was downing six of each, for a total of twelve in each twenty-four hours.

Then suddenly everything started to move through my system in four hours. Panic-stricken, I dropped them altogether for a couple of days. Transit time went up to thirty-six hours.

Well, moderation in all things, I thought. And I went back to a total of five or six a day, colon conditioner and cascara combined. It worked. And I learned a valuable lesson: not only is each person an individual with his own responses, but each individual varies from time to time.

I was about three months into the nutritionist's program when I had to make the above adjustment. Later, I needed less again, and after perhaps a year I was down to only two or three a day. Two years into the program, I dropped them altogether; I simply didn't need them any more. Seven years later, I still take psyllium.

So you can see that you have to experiment with the laxatives for yourself. I know one person who took one cascara capsule—just one—and had diarrhea for three days. That's an unusual case, but it proves a point: individual biochemistry varies a great deal.

Baking Soda Baths Detoxify the Skin

The nutritionist explained that both the bowel and the kidneys are supposed to eliminate a large part of the body's garbage. When these channels don't work as expected, however—and mine most certainly weren't—some of the excess toxins are sent to the lungs and skin for elimination.

I'd never thought of the skin as an organ of elimination.

But it made sense that with both bowel and kidneys overloaded, the skin might try to process some of the body's toxins.

"You need to take soda baths," the nutritionist explained.

"But I already bathe regularly," I objected.

He nodded. "But baking soda draws toxins out of your skin. There's much more to it than just washing the outside."

He went on to tell us how to do it, and from the day he left, I made myself a baking soda soak almost every afternoon. I used a cup and a half of soda in a full tub of water. He said I should stay in it for an hour, warming it up each time it cooled off enough to be comfortable. The idea was to keep sweating, as that helps to flush the toxic material out through the pores of the skin.

He also cautioned me to make the first bath just nicely warm; I could gradually increase the temperature when I was sure it didn't overstimulate my heart. Moreover, someone was to be in the bathroom with me for the duration of each bath for the first week; if I'd happen to faint, he didn't want me drowning in all that water.

As it turned out, I found that if I started each bath with the water just moderately warm and then increased the temperature after I'd been in it for about fifteen minutes, I didn't have any trouble with my heart racing; otherwise, I did.

I'll admit that I was skeptical at first about the baths. What could hot water and baking soda do to detoxify my body? But partway through the very first bath, I began to believe. My skin began to exude waxy, greyish-yellow gunk—greasy stuff that certainly wasn't all dead skin.

I scraped it off with my fingernails and then swished it away with a brush. Going from one area of my body to another, I scraped, though more and more slowly—both the heat and the scraping tired me out—as my hour in the bath wore on.

When at last I'd soaked a full hour, I crawled out gratefully. And crawled is the proper word. I was far too light-headed to stand. I sat on the mat at the edge of the tub for quite a while, first with my head propped against the wall and then with it upright, before I was strong enough to stagger to the bedroom.

I took those soda baths almost daily for many weeks, increasing the temperature whenever the extra heat didn't make my heart race. It must have been a month before the water wasn't murky by the time I was done with it. It was even longer than that until I didn't get the waxy buildup under my nails when I scraped my skin.

So apparently the nutritionist had been right: baking soda dissolved in hot water draws garbage through your skin. No way could all that junk have been stored in my skin though. It, like the colon, must be able to draw toxins from other parts of the body once it's reasonably clean itself.

I still take an occasional soak in soda water; maybe it will prevent a recurrence of toxicity in my skin.

Chapter Twelve

Attogram Candida Purge

When I had earlier been forced to quit nystatin because of the unbearable nausea, I thought the candida and I would have to coexist somehow for however long I lived. I knew the yeast was slowly killing me, but by this point I was too miserable to care.

On his first visit, the nutritionist offered me a natural alternative—a candida killer that didn't make me feel like throwing up for twenty-four hours a day. He was confident that the Attogram Candida Purge could bring my galloping overgrowth under control.

Caprol, the major player in the program, is a solution of caprylic acid in olive oil. It was designed by a pharmacist who had changed to using natural products when drugs had failed him in his own illness.

I was naturally leery of anything designed to kill candida; after my experience with nystatin, I was afraid anything that killed candida would likely about kill me too. But caprylic acid is derived from coconuts, and olive oil could hardly be called a drug. So overall, I couldn't see any reason not to try.

The nutritionist instructed me to take the Caprol mixture

first thing in the morning. That way it would go into my stomach while it was still empty and could get on through quickly. This is important because the mix contains acidophilus, and it's very easily destroyed by stomach acid.

The nutritionist prepared it for me the first morning, and it looked simple enough to do. Just dump all the ingredients into a glass jar, put the lid on, shake it hard for a few seconds, remove the lid, and toss the contents down the hatch. Unless you retch first.

Some people really mind the taste, and others gag over the texture. Neither one bothered me, though I couldn't say I liked it either. But if it had the power to rescue me from the clutches of candida (the nutritionist agreed that candida was my major problem), I felt that I could take it several times a day. After all, if this is going to work, let's get on with it.

"How important is this stuff?" I asked, thinking of those who couldn't manage to get it down.

"Important enough that you won't get well without it," he replied. "This is the heart of the candida control program—and candida is the basis for all your problems. Without this mixture to bring it into line, I don't see how you ever can get well."

His response left me wondering how often I could take the Caprol mixture and how much of it I could handle at a time.

"How rotten can you stand to feel?" he replied when I asked. "You can take as much of it as you can stand. Just don't forget that the more of it you take, the more miserable you'll be!"

I didn't understand his expression at the time. I was already miserable. What did he mean?

Starting on the Mixture

The morning after the nutritionist left after his first visit, I set about mixing the Candida Purge mixture for myself.

"Put ten ounces of water in a jar," I said aloud, only half to my spouse who was standing by. "Now, to add the other ingredients." I picked up the psyllium container and reached for the measuring spoons.

"I thought he told you to add the psyllium last," my long-suffering spouse reminded. "Aren't you to have a hot drink first, too? Then you take the mixture after that."

"Oh, yes! The hot herb tea. I just forgot, that's all."

And so we had our cup of tea. Without sugar, of course. Sugar feeds candida. Caprol kills candida. We were paying for Caprol, so it would hardly make sense to stimulate the candida with sugar.

When our tea was gone, we came back for another round with the Candida Purge.

"I'll put in the bentonite first," I said aloud. "The water's already there." I had lined up all the ingredients on the counter top this time—lined them up in exactly the order the instructions directed to add them to the jar. Hubby's idea, of course: given my foggy mental condition, such a logical notion would never have entered my head.

"Now for the Caprol." I measured it and dumped it in. Next came the acidophilus capsule. I picked it up and started to pull it apart. I held it over the jar in case any of the contents spilled.

Soon the powder was in the jar. So was the longer half of the empty gelatin shell I had shaken it out of. In my concern over the oil-covered piece of capsule floating in the liquid beneath my fingers, I dropped the other half of the shell in too.

"Never mind," my husband advised. "Those things are designed to be swallowed. The only reason the nutritionist had you shake it out was so that it would mix evenly through the rest of the goop."

Casting a jaundiced eye on the Caprol-coated floating capsule halves, I measured the psyllium powder and dumped it in on top. Then I stood there staring at the jar, not sure what to do next.

"Quick! Get the lid on and shake it!" hubby ordered. "The nutritionist said it gets thick and lumpy if you don't take it right away!"

I grabbed the two-pieced home-canning jar lid, plunked it onto the jar, and gave the outer band a speedy twist. My husband was right, of course: that is what the nutritionist had said.

Both pieces of the lid whirled away onto the floor. The flat part landed in the toe space beside the refrigerator and the circluar band came to rest in front of the pantry door.

Hubby retrieved the pieces, and with a grieved expression spun the lid neatly onto the jar. He gave the container a violent shake, and then without spilling a drop he took the lid off again. Holding the jar toward me, he ordered, "Drink it. Now!"

I drank.

It soon became routine, of course. Before too long I could almost go through the whole performance with my eyes shut. But the first time or two it threw me for a loop, which gives ample evidence of the vacant condition of my cotton candy brain.

After we had it down, we drank more tea. Nutritionist's orders, of course. "Warm drinks serve two purposes," he had explained. "They relax the valve at the bottom of the stomach, thus letting the whole mixture pass through as soon as possible. That's important, because stomach acid destroys the acidophilus. Secondly, since psyllium soaks up a lot of fluid, you have to drink extra water so that it doesn't get stuck to your insides."

Accelerating the Program

The only complication I ran into with the Attogram Candida Purge was caused by the hibiscus flowers in the brand of psyllium husk the nutritionist sold. Hibiscus had given me heartburn for years already. So we located some psyllium without hibiscus, and then I could take the mixture without any problem.

And take it I certainly did. I had asked the nutritionist how much I could safely use, and his reply had left me perplexed. But by the end of my third week on the program, I understood his expression when he said, "The more you take, the more miserable you'll feel!"

About the time I had gotten the procedure for mixing the Attogram Candida Purge down pat, I started to increase the amount in every dose. I worked up to the maximum level quickly, then switched from once to several times a day.

Only the first time through was the process really difficult. May I never, however, be found guilty of telling anyone—especially anyone with the brain fag that comes with candida—that it's simple. That first time, it's confusing, to say the least. But it's candida treatment, and it's colon cleansing, and it really must be done.

I did it with a vengeance: a tablespoonful of Caprol, a tablespoonful of liquid bentonite, two acidophilus capsules, and a rounded tablespoonful of psyllium powder at a time—and before more than a month had passed, I was taking those amounts four times a day. (The nutritionist had given me those amounts as the maximum to work up to by the time I was six weeks into the program, and then only once a day.)

Along with the Caprol mixture, I used gallons of water a day—at least four quarts internally plus daily hot soaks in baking soda water. I also swallowed enough cascara sagrada (herbal laxative) and bowel conditioning formula (Nature's Way's Naturalax 2) to push all that bulk through my system in eighteen hours or less.

I would either lick the candida or die while trying.

That Special De-tox Smell

"When I come back six weeks from now, I'll know whether or not you're doing all that I've told you to," the nutritionist warned me as he prepared to leave after his first visit at our house.

"Oh?" I raised my eyebrows. "Will I really have improved that much by then?"

He shook his head. "I'm talking about something else," he said slowly. "The moment I open your door, I'll smell you!"

At first, I thought he had to be teasing me.

"No," he answered. "I meant what I said. When a body harbors as much toxicity as yours does, and you begin to stir things up, the junk escapes in every possible direction. A lot of it will come right through your skin."

It took about three weeks for the smell to develop. By then I could soak for a full hour in a tub of hot baking soda water and within two hours of getting out of it I could smell me too. A close-up sniff of my forearm was enough to make me gag.

The nutritionist had certainly been right; anyone who came near the place could smell me. The aura even went along when my family went away. The entire house, their clothing included, was permeated with the stench.

More than just my skin was discharging garbage. I quickly came to realize that the psyllium does more than just act as a vehicle for the Candida Purge. It also picks up garbage from the colon walls and dumps it along with the regular bowel material.

I was astounded at both the amount and the variety of absolutely awful stuff that started to come from my colon within a few days of starting on the program. This continued, with breaks of anywhere from a few days to a few weeks, for about two years. Some of it was material that had been adhering to my colon wall; some of it, especially as time went on, was garbage that was being drawn into the colon from tissues throughout my body.

I never would have dreamed that so much garbage could have been stored in any one body. Given the amount of it there was, I thought, it's a wonder I hadn't died from the overload.

Thoughts About Water

I want to share some information here about the cheapest "health food" on the face of the earth: water. The adult human body is more than seventy-five percent water; the brain is almost eighty-five percent. The kidneys, colon, lungs, and skin all remove water from the body in the normal course of doing their duty. All this water has to be replaced if the body is to operate at its best.

For example, how can the kidneys filter out the toxic materials that they're supposed to remove from the body if there isn't sufficient water for them to work with? All too often, the kidneys are overburdened because of a shortage of water, and therefore some of the toxic material that should be removed gets stored in your tissues instead; the kidneys simply can't handle it because there's not enough water for them to work with.

The same is true of the lungs: when there's not enough water to go around, the lungs get gummed up with stickier than normal mucus. As a result, lung function is compromised, leading to such serious problems as asthma. (More factors are involved; however, water deprivation is definitely a factor.)

Similarly, many people with stomach and duodenal ulcers find dramatic improvement as they increase the amount of water they drink. This is one of the places that it's especially important to drink a pint of water about thirty minutes before eating. When this is done, the water gets absorbed into the blood stream before food is taken. Then when the stomach begins to call for digestive juices, there's lots of water available to flush them into the stomach. Thus the acid is moved into the volume of food in the stomach instead of remaining at or near the stomach wall where it is produced (and where it may ultimately cause ulcers.)

Then while you are eating, drink very little or no water at all—not more than enough to swallow your supplements. This allows the digestive juices to be maintained at their full strength to digest your food.

Your body needs a minumum of one-half ounce of water per pound of your present weight per day under normal conditions. If you're exposed to a hot, dry environment, or are doing heavy labor, you need more. Perspiration also requires more. In rigorous conditions, you might need as much as an ounce per pound of your weight per day. This level is also desirable when you're undergoing detoxification.

It's a good idea to drink several cups of water first thing in the morning; this flushes the night's accumulated toxins out before the body is again busy with digestion and other daytime activities. If you're on the Candida Purge and use it first thing in the morning, that automatically gives your body a good supply of water to start the day.

Any beverage or medication that contains caffeine acts as a diuretic, drawing fluid out of the body. So for every cup of coffee, tea, or soft drink that contains caffeine, and for every pain pill with it in, drink an extra eight ounces of water to offset the diuretic effect.

Do obtain pure water. The chlorine in town water, for example, is known to destroy the friendly intestinal organisms that normally keep candida under control. Hardly makes sense, does it, to drink it? (You can get rid of most of the chlorine by drawing the water into a pitcher and letting it stand for twenty-four hours; the chlorine volatilizes into the air.)

Fluoride, another ingredient added to drinking water supplies, is known to destroy bone and has other negative effects as well. If you have town water, talk to someone who is knowledgeable about water purifiers, and if necessary, get one and use it. Be cautious, though; many salespeople will make claims for their product that can't be substantiated. Be a knowledgeable consumer by reading up on the subject ahead of time.

Some Alternatives to Caprol

The Attogram Candida Purge consists of several separate components: psyllium, bentonite, acidophilus, and Caprol. The caprylic acid in the Caprol is the actual candida killer. Caprylic acid is also available in tablets and capsules, but these delivery systems are not nearly as effective as Caprol is and they are usually more expensive.

If, for some reason, you must use capsules, open them and mix the contents into the psyllium, etc. If it is a tablet, crush before mixing.

Caprol contains 300 mg of caprylic acid per one-half teaspoon, or 600 mg per teaspoonful. A meaningful therapeutic level might reach 1200 to 1800 mg a day or more. So check your label carefully. Some caprylic acid tablets have only 100 mg each.

At the height of my own candida war, I was using four tablespoons of Caprol a day, dividing it into four doses. That's a total of 7200 mg of caprylic acid a day. I don't recommend that unless you're ready to feel absolutely awful; I certainly did.

This is probably as good a place as any to also clarify the fact that the psyllium in the Candida Purge and the psyllium in the colon cleansing is one and the same. You're not going to use double amounts if you're doing both. Just add the caprylic acid to the psyllium you're using for colon cleansing.

It's also a good place to repeat the warning given in the disclaimer at the beginning of this book: I am telling you of my personal experience; I am not telling you to do what I did.

The appendix includes a referral to the national registry of the Naturopathic Association, including an address and phone number. We recommend that you get professional help if you have problems similar to mine, and the naturopathic route seems to make the best sense of anything we've become aware of.

(As you may remember from the first chapter of this book, the medical world as such—orthodox, or allopathic medicine—had already given me up to die before the nutritionist came. Medicine simply doesn't have anything to offer for problems such as I had. I'd like to think that the day is coming when they will.)

Chapter Thirteen

Cleansers Versus Builders

When the nutritionist interviewed us, we were amazed to find that of all the strange things that were happening in my life, he didn't meet anything new. He did say, however, that he had never been called upon to help any one individual who had nearly all of them at the same time.

My system needed a tremendous amount of help, and by the time he left our house after that first visit I had more pills to take with each meal than I had ever seen anyone swallow at one sitting in my life.

"Think of them as food," he encouraged. "Other than the few cleansers you're taking, this is all just concentrated nutrition done up in tablet and capsule form."

I had driven the poor man almost to distraction at first with my inability to differentiate between cleansers and builders, but by the time he left I had it sorted out. The only cleansers he gave me at that point centered around candida control and colon cleansing. Everything else belonged in the builder group.

There were many of these builders. Kelp capsules, licorice root, adrenal gland substance, alfalfa, burdock, coenzyme

Q-10, pantothenic acid, vitamin B-6, an overall B-Complex, and so on. These supplemental nutrients help the weakened body to regenerate itself. The goal was to rebuild the glands and organs that had degenerated prematurely.

He added digestive enzymes, mainly pancreatin, and stomach acid (betaine hydrochloride) to bolster what I had earlier considered to be a cast iron digestive system. Something about that robust digestion had changed during the last few years, and the system was letting me down with increasing frequency. The almost constant heartburn proved that. So did my terrible intestinal gas and constant burping.

The nutritionist suggested that both the heartburn and the gas traced to a combination of candida overgrowth and poor digestion. Given the amount of gas I was producing, both must have been working overtime. My family had taken to calling me "the lady from Burpees," and recently it wasn't always funny.

I said earlier that nothing really changed in the first three months I followed the nutritionist's program. I'll take that back: both the frequency and the intensity of the heartburn decreased dramatically within a couple of weeks of my beginning to use the digestive aids. I even went back to eating an occasional orange. I had always enjoyed them, but for the past several years I'd had intense heartburn for two or three hours every time I ate one.

(My joy over oranges failed to survive the nutritionist's second visit. He said that I had a very acidic system. Citrus fruit, unless tree ripened, would make the acidity worse.)

No Mineral Pills for Me!

Besides all the herbal and such like builders and the digestive aids, the nutritionist wanted me to use multi-vitamin-mineral tablets as well. Although I had originally set myself to work with him in every way that I conscientiously could, at this point I balked.

The naturopath who had treated me for cancer three years earlier had told us that my liver problems came partly from the DDT and partly from an accumulation of the indigestible part of the mineral pills I'd taken for twenty years.

"There are different forms of calcium and magnesium," he explained. "Some are easy for the body to assimilate and some aren't. Dolomite, oyster shell, eggshell, and the carbonates do contain the minerals, but they're not in anything like food form. Therefore you absorb only a very low percentage of the overall mineral content from these substances.

"Many people excrete the undigested part without any problem," he had gone on to explain. "Obviously, you're one of the people who doesn't. When a person doesn't excrete the undigested minerals, then they're laid down in some inconvenient places in your body. The liver is particularly prone to accumulate them, and once there, they interfere with proper liver function. And that is a part of the reason you have cancer."

He scared me good and proper. Now here was the nutritionist asking me to take the very substances the naturopath had warned me so strongly against. The vitamin-mineral pills he sold contained not only calcium and magnesium carbonate, but di-calcium phosphate as well—another undesirable form of mineral supplement.

I now put my foot down hard about swallowing any more such pills. So the nutritionist and I reached a compromise. I took all his herbal builders and the vitamins, but I stayed away from his mineral supplements. I took half a dozen capsules a day of kelp, alfalfa, and burdock, for a total of eighteen food form units of minerals instead. For trace minerals I took seawater concentrate too, using about two teaspoons a day.

Overall, it worked, though I got tired of swallowing so many extra capsules, especially since I had many others as well.

"I wish someone would marry vitamins and minerals with herbs," I told my husband one day. "I need a product that has higher potencies of minerals than these herbs do but that at the same time is as digestible as they are. That way I could get more nutrients without so many extra pills."

Herbs and Minerals Do Marry

One day about three years after I started onto the nutritionist's program, I was leafing through a magazine from the health food store. There I came across an ad for a supplement that sounded exactly like what I wanted: MegaFood supplements made by Biosan Labs at Derry, New Hampshire. BioMetabolic Nutrition, made by the same company, is exactly the same thing but is the "professional line", and may be carried by your health practitioner. In some states, and with some insurance companies, it might even qualify for reimbursement from your insurer.

If you are in a position to purchase at wholesale, get in touch with them at 1-800-634-6342. For the retail customer, they are available at the health food store. Nutri-Choice, (see Sources in the Appendix), sells this line by mail order at a 35% discount.

The more I learned about the MegaFood products, the better I liked what they were doing. In a nutshell, you might say it as follows: Most multivitamin-mineral pills contain the nutrients in what is known as the U S P form. This is not the form in which the human body uses them, however. So when U S P nutrients are swallowed, the body must then convert them into the proper form for biological utilization. If the person's health is seriously compromised, he might not be capable of making that conversion.

The Biosan company starts with these U S P nutrients, but they don't stop there. Instead, before compressing them into tablets, they put them through a complex series of steps that utilize live plants to turn the U S P nutrients into a form that the human body recognizes as food.

MegaFood and Bio Metabolic Nutrition products have lower stated potencies than many other brands do. But the absorption and utilization by the body is higher. So even though they are more expensive per milligram of a given nutrient, the bottom line is that they're more than worth the difference.

Knowing what I do now, if I couldn't afford Biosan's products, I'd consider taking calcium and magnesium in the citrate forms. This doesn't absorb as well as the MegaFood form, but it's much better than the carbonates, dolomite, oystershell, and so on are.

Lots of Acidophilus

Right from the start, the nutritionist had me using an abundance of acidophilus. This living mocroscopic organism has to be kept refrigerated to maintain its potency. (Those kinds that claim not to need refrigeration don't seem to generally be the strains needed by the human body.)

Acidophilus is available in both powder and capsule form. In general, the capsules are more potent per volume of product, and a better buy. When you go out to buy acidophilus, be cautious; there's a tremendous variation in the number of live organisms per capsule. We've seen anything from twenty million to eight billion. Given that a billion is a thousand million, it would take four hundred of the twenty million capsules to equal one of the eight billion type. So it's definitely a case of let the buyer beware. Anything that can be sold, will be sold, and I suppose that to the uninitiated buyer, twenty million sounds like a great deal.

The nutritionist had me open the acidophilus capsules and mix the contents directly into the Candida Purge. Including them there makes it sound as though they're cleansers. They're not. Acidophilus and other related organisms such as bifidobacterium are builders—the friendly organisms that antibiotics and candida, not to mention birth control pills and sugary foods, have eliminated from the colon.

The acidophilus he gave me contained only lactobacillus. Now I prefer a multistrain product containing both the above and a good portion of bifidobacterium. NOW Foods markets an exceptionally good one, which is called simply 8 Billion Acidophilus and Bifidus. It contains eight billion units, mixed, per capsule. One capsule daily is minimal for a therapeutic effect in an adult; three or four is better. A small child can have one a day; if it's an infant, divide it into several doses. I've often told our daughters to give it to their infants to control diaper rash. It works.

There are certain advantages to mixing the probiotics, as the above items are called, into the Candida Purge combination or at least into some form of bulking agent such as psyllium husk powder.

In the complete Candida Purge, the procedure followed assures that the acidophilus is carried quickly past the stomach (stomach acid destroys probiotics) and on to the intestines, which is where it's needed. An additional advantage of this type of administration is that the bulk created by the psyllium gel spreads the acidophilus into all the folds and crevices of the colon as it passes through.

Lots of Chlorophyll too

Along with the other builders he had me take, the nutritionist insisted that I must have liquid chlorophyll—at least a tablespoonful every day. I took it faithfully for some time, but the mint flavor got to me at last and I gave it up. I did, however, swallow extra capsules of powdered alfalfa juice instead, hoping that since liquid chlorophyll is derived from alfalfa the substitute would be adequate. I've never seen any indication that it wasn't.

Alfalfa juice powder is also available in bulk at a lower cost. And there are other chlorophyll-rich supplements, including chlorella, spirulina, wheat grass powder or tablets, and blue-green algae. I now alternate from one to another of these rather than taking one particular one all the time.

Such green foods are tremendously important, both for prevention of illness and for restoration of wellness. A number of multilevel companies are capitalizing on this fact. Take a close look at their pricing structure and you may find that you'll get a better bargain at the health food store. Or call Nutri-Choice at 715-223-3941 for a mail order source of the NOW Foods line of green foods at a 35% discount.

Dietary Adjustments

Along with the body cleansing and the rebuilding

supplements, the nutritionist immediately emphasized the need to make adjustments to my diet. I had already lived without sweets for about fifteen years, and that was definitely to my advantage. Moreover, we had cut down dramatically on red meat when I was diagnosed with cancer in 1986.

But still the nutritionist wasn't satisfied. On his first visit already, he asked me to consider consuming only the following foods: fruits and vegetables, both raw and cooked (avoiding those too high in carbohydrates); raw nuts and seeds; a little poultry and fish; and lots of raw vegetable juices, with a heavy emphasis on carrot and celery. I could also have a tiny bit of honey.

My husband did all this with me, for he knew that I needed his support if I were to get well. He was probably right, of course: otherwise, I'd not have been able to stick to the diet.

After about six weeks on the new diet, my appetite decreased very greatly all of a sudden. When I called the nutritionist and told him, he suggested that I switch to eating nothing but raw juices and the supplements for several days. I was also to drink lots of water. I maintained this raw juice fast, as he called it, for eleven days before going back to the foods he had outlined when he first came.

We had already been using raw, unrefined flax seed oil since 1986. The particular nutritionist we were working with didn't seem to feel that it was important, but we kept on anyhow. Knowing what we do now, we suspect that I'm not able to convert the L A in flax seed oil into G L A, and that I should have been taking some source of preformed G L A. It was another two and a half years until I began to use borage seed oil capsules for their G L A content, and when I did I had another significant improvement in my health.

Chapter Fourteen

Getting Worse First

The nutritionist had warned me before he came that I'd go backward before I saw improvement. I'd never heard of such a notion, and it didn't make any sense.

Three weeks later, I no longer doubted his word. My condition deteriorated in several ways as I took more and more of his supplements.

My unpleasant body odor increased alarmingly. My energy level took another nose-dive; I came to the point where my body literally didn't want to move. I was so tired that chewing well-cooked food left me worn to a frazzle. Raw veggies were out of the question: I didn't have the energy to eat them.

To add insult to injury, the nutritionist had assigned me extra work. Three or four times a day I mixed and swallowed another batch of the Attogram Candida Purge. I counted out and downed handful after handful of pills. I prepared and cooked and ate half a dozen or more servings of vegetables a day. I made and drank quarts of carrot and celery juices and cleaned up the messy juicer after each use.

Besides all that I did the soda baths. For an hour or more each day I had to soak in a tubful of hot water to which I'd added a cup or more of baking soda. This, the nutritionist said, would draw out some of the toxins through my skin, thus making less burden on the other eliminative organs.

He was certainly right about the toxins; I must have done those daily baths for almost a month before the water would still be clear when I got back out of it. My skin literally oozed garbage, and all the while I was soaking I'd keep scraping away at it with my fingernails, covering my whole body several times over in the course of each hour-long bath. I left my fingernails long on purpose, and as I scraped, they would fill up with gunk. I'd clean it out with a brush every little while and then start scraping again.

I guess it's no wonder I laid the blame for my lowered energy level on the nutritionist. If he hadn't given me the extra work, I wouldn't be so tired. About the third time I said so to my husband, he gently reminded me that the nutritionist could hardly derive any satisfaction from loading me with work. Moreover, hadn't he given me fair warning? He told me before he ever came that I'd get worse before I began to feel better.

Well, I guess. But why did I have to feel so very rotten? If these herbs-and-nutrition people were so smart, why couldn't they devise some system whereby a sick person didn't have to get worse before he could get better?

And then I remembered the look on the nutritionist's face the moment I had asked him how often it would be all right to use the Attogram Candida Purge. It was true enough; he had been fair.

When I realized why I felt as awful as I did, I almost decided to back down; to revert to taking the mixture just once a day. Further thought, however, convinced me to persist. Although I didn't exactly like the changes I'd seen so far, at least there had been changes. Given the volume of garbage my body kept eliminating, my condition almost had to improve before too long.

Emotional Upheaval

When the weeks continued to go by and I didn't get well, I

almost gave up in despair. I wasn't going to get better after all. Sometimes in spite of my best intentions, I would give way to tears. The following incident illustrates this.

The crunch of tires on hard-packed snow came to me from the driveway as I watched my family leave for church.

"Can't go! Can't go! Can't go!" Like a pronouncement of doom, the cadence of the tires mocked my hurting spirit, and the echo in my consciousness mimicked the refrain: "Can't go! Can't go! Can't go!"

The sobs I'd been biting back for the past half-hour came freely now. Disconsolate, I slumped into a chair and gave myself without restraint to my grief.

When I first became so allergic to chemicals that I couldn't circulate in society anymore, I had supposed that even a people-oriented person like me would eventually become accustomed to staying at home when my husband and our daughters went away. But week after week had plodded by, and still each departure brought an emotional storm.

Permission to Grieve

I called it self-pity at first, and despised my weakness. Then an article by L.M. Marshall, M D, helped to ease my guilt about the tears. He encouraged those who had lost their health to cry about it if they could, for loss of health is devastating, and the victim needs to go through a period of mourning. Crying can be a very effective release.

A period of mourning. I hadn't thought of it that way before. Thank you, Dr. Marshall, whoever and where ever you are, for permission to cry. To mourn the loss of something precious even though it isn't another person.

I had faced bereavement in the past, and had known the almost despairing sense of personal loss that comes when a loved one dies. But I had wept for those who were gone, and even more for myself because I missed them, and gradually the raw edges of the pain were soothed while acceptance took the place of anguished sorrow.

Permission to think of my loss of health as being a form of

bereavement now allowed me to apply the grieving process to this loss as I had to the others. I also began to realize that there was more involved. When a person dies, others gradually come to take the place, at least in some measure, of the one who is no longer there, and after a while the initial void gives way to ongoing life.

Losing my health was entirely different in that respect, however. The nature of my illness—the fact that I could no longer be with other people because the scented personal care items they used cut off my breathing—left me unable to circulate in society at all. Therefore people could not fill the vacuum in my life.

The freedom to grieve didn't help me to get well physically, but it did make it possible for me to cope more effectively with the circumstances of my existence. It helped me to maintain whatever degree of sanity I still had during those months when I could see no reason to hope that I would ever be well again. It bridged the gap until the food supplements, body detoxification, hormone balancing, diet changes, and other lifestyle adjustments had a chance to bring some degree of recovery onto my horizon.

I Am Thankful

I'm thankful now for the victories that I gained in my overall health picture as a result of the nutritionist's program. The healing process, however, is still incomplete, being hindered by several irreversible factors that trace to my childhood.

Repeated inhalation of D D T for a number of years while I was very young. Massive doses of antibiotics when I had rheumatic fever at age seven. Poor diet throughout my growing years. The merciless way I drove my unwilling body during my teens and twenties. Each has contributed its share to the limits that seem to have been set on my getting well.

But as I said, I'm thankful for all the improvements. There are still occasions, however, when I'm grateful for the release of pent-up emotions that can come through guilt-free tears.

Chapter Fifteen

This is Progress?

The second time the nutritionist came, he said I'd made wonderful progress. He also left five hundred dollars worth of assorted supplements for me to take. (Six weeks earlier, on his first visit, the bill had been about six hundred and fifty dollars.)

By the time of his second visit, I had begun to suspect that nothing was going to happen. Other than the disappearance of my constant heartburn, I'd seen no improvement. Nothing. Meanwhile, I not only felt more awful than I had at the start; now I smelled awful too.

I never did see any parasites such as the books the nutritionist had left with us described. He had told me already on his first visit that they weren't a part of my problem, though as he said, he couldn't for the life of him figure out why I didn't have them. Well, I had enough other garbage stored in my system to more than compensate for the absence of a few little parasites.

At this point, my colon was still discharging foul-smelling junk frequently and in remarkable amounts.

"Wonderful!" the nutritionist enthused when I told him so. "The more of those toxins we're able to get out of your system, the better chance you have of getting well!"

But I had already been on his program for six weeks. I was still swallowing more than a hundred assorted pills a day plus several powders and liquid preparations. And so far I hadn't seen a shred of evidence that anything would ever improve.

My colon was cleansing; of that there was no doubt. But nothing else had improved except the heartburn. At his first visit already he had intimated that I might be better in three months. (Not until later did he tell me that in cases as severe as mine it always takes longer than that.)

I did already know that it takes at least a year to thoroughly cleanse the average North American's colon. I also knew that additional cleansing is needed to regulate the liver, the blood, and the tissues. I was looking forward to getting on with these. I didn't know that as the colon cleansing progresses, some of the toxins that have been in storage throughout the body begin to move into the circulation. From there, they're dumped into the colon for elimination. This happens even though the person isn't using products specifically designed to cleanse any other organ than the colon.

When these stored poisons start to come out into the circulation, they can make you feel worse than you did while they were being held in the tissues. This is because they travel through the blood stream and the blood stream goes through the brain. In spite of the blood-brain barrier, some of these liberated poisons get into your brain tissues, making you feel really rotten.

So you can see that this rotten feeling is a part of the price of a cleaner, more efficient body. Ultimately, when the toxins are gone, you'll feel better than you have for a very long time. Unless, of course, you have other imbalances that also need to be corrected.

The nutritionist never mentioned the fact, but we later learned that if the toxin level in the blood stream gets too high, it can cause an elevated heart rate. So if you're cleansing, monitor your resting heart rate to be sure it doesn't go too high. (Consult your personal health care provider to determine what is too high for you.)

I didn't know about heart rate monitoring while I was cleansing heavily, so I have no idea whether mine increased. I do know that my body was getting cleaner. It had to be. Later on I learned that until the colon is reasonably clean you never feel as though you've improved. It's no real marvel I wondered if *this* is progress.

The Stench Continues

As time went on and no good changes appeared, my family began to express some hesitation.

"It isn't working, is it?" one of my sisters asked. "In spite of everything you're doing, you aren't getting better."

"Not that I can tell," I had to admit. "I keep eliminating lots of garbage, but so far as the actual symptoms go, nothing but the heartburn seems to have changed."

My visitor wrinkled her nose. "The atmosphere is different from earlier," she said. "Did he give you a clue how long the stench might last?"

She could have been more discreet, but she had a valid point about the smell. It wasn't just the body odor any more; I had also started to pass foul smelling gas in such abundance that the odor permeated the house and everything in it. I didn't know why at the time. I'd had gas for years, but nothing that smelled like this. The stench *was* awful.

All the nutritionist knew was that the smell goes with cleansing when the patient is as ill as I had been. Later, we learned more.

The normal acidity level of the intestines is about 6.5. With my sort of problems, it often gets up into the range of 7.8 to 8. As the person cleanses and the body becomes more balanced, the balance between alkaline and acid begins to move toward normal again.

All of this is fine except for the fact that the worst-smelling gas is produced at about 7.2 acidity. And how can you get from 7.8 to 6.5 without passing 7.2?

I suppose this is one of the best (or is that one of the worst?)

illustrations I know of to show that in the process of getting better, temporarily we might get worse instead.

The Sugar Monster Yields to Adrenal Rebuilding

I had lived with a desperate sugar hunger for sixteen years before the nutritionist came on the scene. For many years already, though, the treat that sweets gave my tastebuds cost me more in misery than I was willing to pay. So I had consistently gone without.

But the craving—the terrible sugar hunger—had never gone away. Even today (1996), after having done much serious work on the underlying causes of the craving, I'll often eat far more sweets than I ought to if I take a single bite.

But it's easier now to leave them alone, for in 1990 we learned from the nutritionist how to rebuild the adrenal glands. These glands modulate sugar cravings as well as the desire for starches.

Specifically for the adrenals, I used 600 mcg of chromium picolinate, 4 licorice root capsules, 1,000 mg of pantothenic acid (that's vitamin B-5), 6 kelp capsules (not the tablets), a tablespoonful of cold-pressed, unrefined flaxseed oil, 3,000 mg of vitamin C (ester C form), several capsules of vitamin B complex, and a combination of herbs specifically designed for the adrenals (ADR-NL from Nature's Way).

We have since learned that some people, myself apparently included, benefit by also using borage seed oil capsules, usually two per day. (Borage is pretty potent; it's best to start with half a capsule a day, and work up gradually.)

Also, women with compromised adrenals often get a lot of benefit by using natural progesterone. It's available in skin cream form for transdermal (through the skin) administration.

There are many products on today's market. Some of them are purely wild yam extract, and your body has to convert the diosgenin in them to progesterone. If it can, this is our preferred route.

Others contain U S P progesterone, which is easier for the

compromised biochemistry to utilize. One that contains actual progesterone is called Pro-Gest, and is sold by Sedna (see appendix).

The natural progesterone products help to regulate female-system hormone imbalances, including PMS. They also contribute directly to adrenal gland repair, for progesterone is the precursor molecule at least for many of the adrenal hormones.

I personally didn't learn about natural progesterone until the summer of 1992. I began to use it generously right away, and within about two months, my gross PMS came under almost complete control. In addition, many of my other symptoms underwent further improvement. I still use it, though not nearly as often as I did then.

Getting the adrenals back into shape also requires much rest—at least eight hours each night plus a good nap in the afternoon. It's also wise to take frequent brief periods of total relaxation during the course of the day. I recommend ten minutes out of each two hours.

During these breaks, you must relax as completely as you can. Concentrate on letting go of the tension in your jaw, around your eyes, and in the roof of your mouth. It may help to massage these areas. This lets your entire body relax amazingly well.

The adrenal rebuilding process made a dramatic difference in my life. Among the changes was a greater ability to cope with emergencies, better tolerance for bright sunshine, the disappearance of the tendency to faint when arising quickly from a prone or squatting posture, and most blessedly of all, the lessening of the craving for sweets.

Earlier, I had avoided them because they put me flat on my back unable to move or make a sound for twenty minutes at a time. Now, with stronger adrenals, I can usually walk away from them because I no longer crave them. (Also, I no longer get the dramatic negative reaction when I do use them, though if I eat much, I'll feel groggy afterward.)

I never make something sweet for myself anymore. But even now, one bite, especially if taken when I'm hungry, can start a binge. I guess I really am a sugarholic.

Apnea: Failure to Breathe

This seems to be the only logical place to discuss apnea, which is the failure of the breathing reflex to function properly. I didn't learn that this particular symptom had a name until I hardly ever had it anymore. I also didn't know until it was about gone that it's a direct result of weak adrenal function.

My apnea developed gradually, and I had it for many years. The more relaxed I was, the more likely it was to strike. Most often of all it came during the night. I'd wake up with a start, gasping for air and feeling as though someone was tightening a steel band around my chest.

After a few seconds of struggling to get started, I'd begin to breathe again. Sometimes I'd have to stay awake and consciously regulate my respiration for a while, or I'd stop breathing again.

I got it during the day as well, though not often. I'd just suddenly realize that I wasn't breathing. Sometimes it would take several hours of consciously regulating my breathing before the reflex would kick in again.

Looking back, I realize that as I recovered from the other symptoms of adrenal exhaustion, the apnea kept pace. As of the present writing, it hardly ever strikes anymore. If it does, I can about guarantee that I'm in the presence of chemicals that I don't detect otherwise. Either that or I've eaten too much sugar.

Chapter Sixteen

Visit Number Three

My family stuck by me in spite of the smell, and was there when the nutritionist came for his third encounter. I'd been on his program for three months by then. If my problem with chemicals had improved at all during that time—and he had come because of my problem with chemicals—the alteration had been too small to detect.

At this point, I still hadn't learned to think of arrested negative motion as improvement. When a problem that's been getting progressively worse slows down and then comes to a standstill, it's a very positive sign. I realized this later on. But when I was in the midst of my many difficulties, and especially the exquisitely tuned sensitivity to chemicals, no actual improvement looked like nothing happening.

The nutritionist had told me on his first visit already that it would be three months till I saw improvement. Well, I did have to admit now that I was occasionally able to detect a little spark of initiative again—and initiative had been conspicuously missing for quite a number of months.

There had also been an almost imperceptible improvement in the brain fag—the awful mental confusion and exhaustion—

though I still thought of myself as having a cotton candy brain.

But as far as the chemical problem went, I hadn't seen a whisper of improvement.

"You Will Get Better"

"You're better, at least," the nutritionist insisted when he came this time. "No one knows if you'll ever get truly well. We don't even know how much you can improve."

"O.K.," I answered. "I think I'm beginning to understand. I'm too impatient."

He grinned. "I wouldn't want to say that," he said. "And I guess I did lead you on a bit at the first there when I told you that you'd be better in three months. I knew you had no way of knowing what to expect. I also knew that if I told you the truth, you wouldn't have even tried to get well. So maybe I did stretch the facts a bit, but my motive was good. And actually, some people do get better in as little as six weeks."

"Not with problems like mine, they don't!" I shot back. "There's no way you can make me believe that!"

He nodded. "Given your problems, no one sees improvement in six weeks. When it doesn't come in that time frame, the changes usually start at about six months. It either takes six weeks or else half a year."

"For everyone?" I asked.

"No and yes. Cases like yours are always half a year—often more. Other than a gross elimination of toxins, they don't see very much change before six months."

"So I shouldn't expect improvement for at least another three months then?" I asked.

"Well, maybe." He wrinkled his forehead. "You've taken heavier doses than I recommend, you know. As much as you've used of both the builders and the cleansers, I think some of your symptoms should turn around before long. With all the stuff you've taken, you deserve it!"

"So what changes might I expect?" He had me curious now.

"Your energy level will begin to improve," he answered. "And I hope that by the next time I come—you'll have been on the program for almost five months by then—we'll see a change in the brain fag too. Pretty soon now, you're going to start to think."

"It's already easing off," I admitted. "I'd forgotten to tell you—you can see it's not much of an improvement yet!—but I think I remember things a little better than I did. Just in the last week, for instance, I'm really starting to retain some of the information I read in those books I bought from you the first time you were here."

"See!" he exclaimed. "I told you to give it time and it would improve!" He grinned as he went on. "I think you'll see a lot of changes by the time you've been at it six months. Even with imbalances as serious as yours."

"Why doesn't everyone get into the kind of trouble I did?" I asked next. "Why do I have all these problems, chemical sensitivity included, while others go scot free?"

He shrugged. "Heredity partly: you have a weak constitution. The D D T exposures when you were very young. Weakened glands. Poor digestion. All those antibiotics over the years. The chemicals in the superinsulated house you lived in a dozen years ago. The tremendous candida overgrowth in your system. It all adds up.

"But at this point, for you, it's not so important what caused your problems. The point now is, what can you do about them?"

I could accept that. But I wasn't done with him yet on the timing score. "Are you ready now to tell me what's actually going to happen?" I challenged. "How soon will I get over the sensitivity to chemicals?"

He shrugged. "How would I know. Two years from now, it won't be nearly as bad as it is now. By then, you'll have made a tremendous amount of improvement."

Two years? I felt my shoulders sag. The nutritionist sat there while I cried, waiting to speak until I had dried my tears.

"I see I shouldn't have told you that," he said then. "I'm sorry. From the way you were talking, I thought you were ready for it. I should have known better. This always comes as a big disappointment. But you have to realize that you didn't get into this condition overnight. With a problem of twenty years duration, you need at least two years of intensive treatment to reach the maximum level of improvement you're capable of attaining. Beyond that, I truly don't know."

Plodding On

And so I took courage, partly from the tiny bits of improvement I'd seen so far, and partly from the nutritionist's assurance that if I had patience, more changes would follow.

At least he seemed pretty sure that I'd get my energy back. And he was really optimistic about my brain function. If those two factors returned to normal, I thought, I'd be a long way ahead of the level at which I had existed for the last six months before he had come onto the scene.

With a functional brain and some energy, I should be of use for something anyhow. Maybe it wouldn't matter so much that I couldn't circulate freely in society. At least there would be something for me to do that I could handle. Some purpose for my being in this world.

So I committed myself to carry on, taking all the supplements even though I saw precious little results.

Something for my Liver

When the nutritionist was with us this time (his third visit), he finally decided that I was ready to start something for my underactive, overworked, clogged-up liver. "I told you from the start that you'd have to wait three months," he said. "You had to cleanse the colon first."

"But the colon cleansing isn't done," I countered. "I'm still dumping horrendous amounts of really ugly garbage. Could I be ready for a liver program yet?"

I didn't come right out and tell him so, but I had played the part of the brave girl long enough. I was tired of feeling rotten all the time. Now that my prospects had begun to look up, I was eager for more improvement. If he gave me something for my liver now, might it mean more misery again? I'd rather finish the colon cleansing first. Future heroics could be left to someone else.

The nutritionist frowned at my reluctance. "I think you're ready now," he said. "As hard as you've gone at the colon cleansers and the builders, and as long as it's been since you started on the program, I'm ready to give you something for your liver."

He must have read the hesitation I was feeling, for his tone became more gentle as he went on. "We won't do anything but silymarin for now. It's more subtle than some of the liver things are. But don't think it isn't effective. It is."

So I began taking silymarin, using three or four capsules a day. (Knowing more about it now, I recommend starting with one a day and gradually working up to four or six.)

At first I couldn't tell any difference from using silymarin. But within a week or so I started to understand what the nutritionist had meant on his first visit, when he had told me how bad liver cleansing can make you feel. And silymarin is more of a builder than it is a cleanser. It sure made me wonder what liver cleansers would have done to me right at the start.

The silymarin was added to everything else I'd already been doing. That was how the nutritionist operated: start with something, do it a while, then add something to it. At no point during the time I worked with him did he ever suggest substituting something for something else. It was always add, add, add.

And so it was that several weeks after I'd started the silymarin he told me it was time for the more aggressive liver herbs to be added. He put me on six capsules daily of each of burdock and dandelion root. There was also a choline, inositol, and methionine mixture. I don't remember at all how much of it I took.

I felt worse again, of course. But the amount of garbage I was dumping from the bowel increased again, which I now knew indicated that I was "making wonderful progress."

When I felt worse this time, therefore, I tried to be optimistic. My whole body was toxic, and those poisons had to come out before I could recover. I understood that now. So even though I felt worse again, I stayed on the liver cleansers.

Blood Purifiers at Last

Several weeks later again, the nutritionist finally gave me the green light for blood purifiers. Red clover combination, echinacea, and a mixture of bugleweed and yellow dock were all added to my seemingly endless list of supplements. By this time, my "fix" was costing us about ten or twelve dollars a day. Fortunately, we could afford it.

We later learned about sources of supplements that offer quality products at much lower prices. In the appendix of this book we will refer you to some of them. Do be cautious, though; not all supplements are equal, and especially if you're very ill, you do need good quality.

On the other hand, it isn't necessary to go to extremes to locate the very best. Only in rare cases is one product really noticeably superior to most others on the market. So if someone—especially someone who sells supplements—tells you that one particular company's products are superior to all others, well, probably not.

The nutritionist did have me start into the blood purifiers slowly. That's always wise, especially with cleansers. We now recommend beginning with only one of the above, and taking just one capsule of it each day at first. Increase every few days. A maximum level would be about four each of the red clover combo and the echinacea, and two a day of the bugleweed-yellow dock type. It's better to take them for a prolonged time than to load up on too many at once.

Chapter Seventeen

Improvement Begins

The nutritionist was right; I continued to improve. Gradually at first, then more rapidly, my energy returned. My thinking cleared. And finally, five and a half months after I began to work with him, I saw the first indication that the chemical problem might yield at least to some extent—and the chemical problem had been my major concern right from the beginning.

I'll likely always remember the first indication of improvement in my level of sensitivity. Someone opened the door of our wood-burning stove. I was sitting on the opposite side of the room and I saw a wisp of smoke escape from the firebox.

When I saw that smoke, I knew I'd have to go for fresh air soon. But being lazy at the time, I decided to wait until it reached me before I'd move. Within a few seconds I could smell smoke. I was about to get up when I realized that I was still breathing freely in spite of the smell.

It was the first time in more than two years that I'd been able to breathe in the presence of enough smoke that I could smell it. I cried, of course, for during my months of treatment

I had hoped and then given up so many times. Now I hardly knew whether or not I dared to believe that some day I would again have some degree of victory over the monster that had plagued me for so long.

Gradually I noticed other changes. The fumes from the blender motor no longer stopped my breathing. Nor did the presence of a person or two wearing clothing that had been washed in scented laundry powder. (I still couldn't be in a crowd; I still can't.)

I didn't experience any sudden changes; the whole healing procedure was a gradual uphill climb—a series of advances and regressions that would have totally perplexed me had the nutritionist not warned me in advance that it would work that way. And as he had said, each advance left me at a higher level of recovery than I had attained before. Consistent with this, each regression didn't drag me quite so far down either.

Because I had such major imbalances to start with, it was possible for me to improve dramatically and still look to those who hadn't known me at the peak of my sensitivities as though I was still acutely ill. Even today, seven years after we began with the nutritionist, I can't mingle into a crowd. The cumulative effect of the fragrances tightens up my chest and stops my breathing.

I can, however, function on the fringes of the crowd. And that's a tremendous improvement over my condition when the nutritionist first came.

For the sake of understanding on the part of those who sincerely believed that spiritual problems underlaid my physical symptoms, I can only say that to the best of my knowledge no spiritual renewal either preceded or accompanied my recovery. It really does seem we were dealing with a physical problem.

I certainly thank the Lord for the improvements!

Progress Continues

The changes came so slowly that at times I had to remind myself how seriously ill I'd been; otherwise I hardly noticed that I was getting well. I had a little strength and endurance again. My thinking was much clearer, though it was still hard to learn new things.

Short-term memory gradually returned. The terrible tiredness wasn't so overpowering any more. I'd started into treatment sleeping fourteen hours of each twenty-four. Now I was down to nine or ten. (Later on, it dropped again; now I need eight or nine.)

So step by step, I began to regain normal functioning. I kept on taking all the builders the nutritionist had recommended, of course. I couldn't expect continuing improvement if I were to stop doing the things that had initiated the changes.

I also continued on the cleansers and the diet. These too, I knew, had contributed immensely to my healing. Why would I want to change them now?

Fasting for More Improvement

The first partial fast I did is detailed earlier in this book. That time, I stayed on the restricted program for eleven days. During the fast and for some time after it was over, I could tell that I was eliminating more garbage than I'd been before I started it.

During the following three years, I fasted several times to promote further cleansing. At first I did the partial fast; I'd drink raw vegetable juices and take supplements, but completely avoid solid foods.

Later I worked through several sessions with nothing but water (not even the cleansers), keeping it up for anywhere from a week to ten days at a time. I did this about once every three months for quite a while.

Between fasting sessions I still ate only vegetables, fruits, nuts and seeds (raw), some whole grains, and a bit of fish or poultry.

The elimination of garbage gradually lessened even during fasting, and three years after I started with the program it finally stopped altogether. About this time I found that I no longer needed laxatives. But I still continue to use the psyllium-based fiber mixture and I keep my water intake very high.

At least one week out of each month I take Attogram's Candida Purge as well. I also routinely use a maintenance intake of a wide spectrum of builders, including several digestive aids, a number of green foods, flax and borage seed oils, Co Q-10, grape seed antioxidant, vitamin B Complex, pantothenic acid, ester C, zinc, chromium, natural beta carotene, Bio Metabolic's Bio Max multiple (same as MegaFood's Alpha), and so on. I also use the natural progesterone cream about one third of the time.

I do all these things without knowing whether or not I really need to. I never want to go back to where I was before the nutritionist came.

There are two reasons for that. The first is simply that I'd rather be dead than live in that state again. The second is that with many people who have been desperately ill, a second return to wellness is much more difficult—and in some cases, impossible—to attain. I don't know why, but it sometimes works that way. It's a chance I'm just not willing to take.

A Word of Warning

Please note that the above is a list of the supplements I use. It is not a set of recommendations for you. I neither diagnose other people's ills nor prescribe what they should do about them. That must be between you and your health care adviser.

In Retrospect

Sometimes we fail to appreciate the forest because the tree in front of our faces prevents us from seeing the whole. This can happen in the alternative health care field as anywhere else. Knowing all we do now, we can see that the nutritionist who helped me so much had his imbalances too—imbalances in his emphases on the causes and what is needed for recovery.

Take, for instance, his almost fanatical concentration on

the candida overgrowth. It's not that it didn't need to be brought under control; I never would have recovered unless it was. But we now know that there was more than just candida overgrowth and body toxicity at the root of my problems.

While the nutritionist mentioned some of these other imbalances (thyroid inadequacy, for instance) he didn't really do as much about them as he could have. Nor did he do anything specific for the female hormone disregulation. All these things, he felt, would fall into place when the candida came under control.

Well, yes and no. Maybe for some people they do. For me, they didn't. (See the following section for some details.) So while we are grateful for all he did for us, we do feel now that my recovery could have been at least somewhat faster had he been aware of more of the needs of my body and what to do for them. But at least his treatment gave me back my brain, and with that I could pursue further details on my own. The literature is there; one just needs to read it and then apply what he has read.

The error of blaming so many symptoms on just a couple of causes (in my case, candida overgrowth and body toxicity) is common. Different practitioners focus on different things, so please be cautious when you look for an adviser. Let's suppose that you have a number of strange symptoms—perhaps symptoms for which your medical doctor would refer you for psychiatric care. Now suppose that you consult a nutrition-oriented adviser.

Whether he beams his spotlight on candida or body toxicity, parasites or vitamin deficiencies, adrenal weakness or the need for nutritional oils, be very slow to believe that all your symptoms are traceable to just one or two underlying problems. More than likely, a number of factors have become unbalanced. You'll regain your health much more quickly and completely by addressing all of them.

As indicated in my history, it isn't always wise or even possible to do everything at once. There is a proper sequence. But in the end, everything must be done that needs to be done.

Proceed with caution, of course. But you must proceed. And you must address everything that needs to be addressed. Otherwise, you'll end up spending a lot of money but will never become as well as you could have had you been more thorough.

Borage Seed Oil and Natural Progesterone

About two and a half years after the nutritionist came on the scene, we learned how unlikely it is for someone with my degree of health problems to convert the L A of flax seed oil to G L A. The body needs both, and there aren't any sources of preformed G L A in our ordinary food.

When we learned that, we added borage seed oil to my line of supplements. So far as we can tell, it is the most economical source of G L A. It's potent stuff, though, so it might be best to start with just half a capsule each day. I worked up to four a day for a while, then backed down to two. Even one a day goes a long way.

I started using the natural, herb-source progesterone in a skin cream form at exactly the same time as I began the borage seed oil. Therefore, I can't prove which did the most for me, or whether the combination did the trick. But I saw improvement in many ways within six weeks of starting these two additional items.

My P M S had cleared by perhaps twenty percent in the first two and a half years of taking the supplements the nutritionist recommended. But it took a very decided turn for the better about six weeks after I started the borage seed oil and the Pro-Gest cream. Within a few months I experienced about a ninety percent improvement. At the same time my tolerance of chemicals got noticeably better again. And it's stayed better since. (I still use the supplements, of course.) This change in the sensitivity to chemicals was a bonus at this point; I'd not thought of the possibility of these things helping that.

Had I used these two items from the beginning of my nutritional program, might I have seen improvement more quickly back then? We suspect I would have, but of course we'll never know for sure.

No Carbon Copies

You need to understand that I'm not telling you what will work for you. There are no biochemical carbon copies, and your body is truly unique. Experimentation is the route to discovery.

As long as you stay with the builders, starting with small amounts and increasing them gradually, and staying within reasonable limits (people who work in health food stores should know what reasonable limits are), you shouldn't have any problem with them. Just don't get in a hurry. And remember that unless you use a decent diet, the pills won't likely be able to do what's needing done.

Above all, don't fall into the trap of "one pill for one ill", and take huge amounts of something, even if it's something good. The one-pill-at-a-time approach makes sense with drugs; it's just as well not to mix too many of them together anyhow. You could create a Pandora's box indeed!

Many of the experts in the supplement field feel, and probably rightly so, that the chances of making a significant impact with nutrients is much enhanced by using several of them together. After all, they're just food, and we don't hesitate to combine carrot sticks with a hamburger. One practitioner, a professional medical man who has turned to the natural route to help his patients, refers to his system as kitchen sink medicine. He claims that the more of the possibly applicable substances you use at once, the greater the probability of improving the patient's condition. His kitchen sink reference, of course, goes back to the idiom "everything but the kitchen sink."

There Isn't Any Magic

There really isn't. You must eat wisely. You must rest enough. You must drink plenty of water. You must live in harmony with your conscience. If you do not do these things, then swallowing a bunch of pills, no matter how good they are, won't do the job you're wanting done. You have to do it all at once, too. It won' t work piecemeal.

Even then, it may take a long time to see results. A few weeks isn't a fair trial when you're working with nutritional substances. Your body must be helped to overcome the effects of years of deficiencies—or in the case of cleansers, years of excesses.

Remember, too, that the supplements aren't medicine; they're food. Therefore the quantities of pills required will seem almost incredibly large. No one would ever take that much medicine. That's all right; these things aren't medicine, they're food.

Compensating for the Past

I have spent several thousands of dollars on supplements over the past seven years. We never kept track of the actual amount. At the moment I take somewhere between two and three dollars worth per day. I'll likely continue to do so—I have to make up for the past.

I'm not addicted to these things; you don't get addicted to them. But my compromised body needs the supplemental nutrients in order to function at its best. I was a very long way down. I never want to go anywhere near to that condition again.

The experts are generally agreed that it sometimes takes as much as ten times the amount of any given nutrient to make you well again as it would have taken to have kept you well in the first place. We not only have to make up for past deficiencies; we also have to repair the damage caused by the shortage of these nutrients in our systems over the years. A motor overhaul costs more than regular oil changes do.

It's similar with cleansing. If I had eaten a high-fiber diet all along and had taken in plenty of water, I wouldn't have built up the body toxicity that I did. I also shouldn't have eaten nearly so much meat as I did; much body toxicity consists of improperly digested particles of meat stored in the tissues.

Once the toxicity is established, however—once the tissues are infiltrated with stored poisons—it takes more than an ordinary high-fiber diet to get it out again. You have to use supplemental fiber consistently and over a long period of time, or the toxins just won't move.

You also have to use liver purifiers like burdock, dandelion, and the choline, inositol, and methione combination as well as liver builders like silymarin. These get the liver cleansed and rebuilt.

Then come the blood-and-tissue-purifying herbs such as echinacea and red clover combination. And of course you have to take lots of herbal laxatives to keep all that garbage moving out of the body. If you don't, a lot of it will get reabsorbed back into the blood stream while it's sitting in the colon waiting to be evacuated.

All these things have to be done in their proper order. See chapter eleven and onward in this book for that information. It's a long, slow, sometimes discouraging process, but as the nutritionist told us when he first came, if I knew of an easier way, I sure would tell you.

Chapter Eighteen

Will Anybody Listen?

The scars on my spirit don't fester any more, and I've come to grips with the memory of rejection and its pain. Now I hurt in a different way, though it too leaves me feeling helpless and tempted to frustration. For around me I see people starting blithely down the path I've already walked.

They're not so far along as I was when things got bad—not yet. But they've begun the downward slide toward full-blown environmental illness with its resultant mysteries and misunderstandings. Neither they nor the people around them have a clue as to what's happening, but though they do not understand it, the monster inside of them ever grows. If all the right circumstances arrive together—and amazingly often they do—that monster will someday attack them with a fury beyond their most vivid imagination.

How can I warn them to change their course in time? How can I compel them to believe that the horrors I experienced were very real and very awful? How can I convince them that they or someone they love might meet similar circumstances in the future? Similar or worse?

How can I persuade young parents—and some who aren't

so young—of the dangers to their precious children of repeated antibiotics for ear infections (most of which are caused by an allergy to the cow's milk that either they or their nursing mothers are drinking), colds, and the flu? How can I help them to see what might be waiting for their offspring at the end of the antibiotic road? (Many of my problems were caused by antibiotics.) How can I constrain them to believe?

Even more difficult, how can I help them to understand the foolhardiness of feeding their little ones a diet that's loaded with sugar and white flour and the things made from them? This includes artificially fruit-flavored "juices" and all forms of candy and other such foodless foods. How can I convince them that for some of these precious little ones, such substances will set the stage for a nightmare of untold horrors in the future? Horrors that they as parents have never dreamed of?

From personal experience, I know. I've been well nigh to the end of that road myself. My family and I have lived through a twofold nightmare—my illness plus the almost total lack of acceptance it generated among our friends and families—for quite a number of years.

Does anybody out there want to listen?

Do You Fit Here Somewhere?

You must have some personal interest in the subject of this book, or you wouldn't have read this far. The story isn't compelling enough to hold the attention of someone who doesn't experience some personal involvement, either directly or on behalf of somebody they love.

I feel that there are three groups of people who should read and heed the story I have told. They are described below.

Group One

These are the people who are already responding negatively to chemicals. By association, it also includes those dedicated folks who stand by them, come what might. Let me assure you that you are not alone. Depending upon the degree of your sensitivity, tens or even hundreds of thousands of people share your fate.

In North America today, more than ten thousand people are unable to circulate in society at all. Many times ten thousand more follow not far behind.

I want this book to reassure you and those around you that your troubles are based upon physical imbalances and are not the product of your imagination. I also hope that I've been able to help you to understand that there is an answer—that you aren't doomed for life to being a recluse, a social leper with weird symptoms no one has heard of, and that therefore must be all in your head.

I also want to fling out a warning to those tens of thousands who are about to follow to the place where you are now. Please, folks, take my word for it: when you get there, you will not be where you were wanting to go.

Group Two

My second audience is those who now stand at the threshold of that door on which is written "Environmental Sensitivity: Untold Horrors Ahead." How can I help these blithely unconcerned people to realize the far-reaching effects of the choice that is before them? There is no neutral ground. Anyone with sensitivity to chemicals will, if he lives for very long, develop more-acute sensitivities. He will also begin to react to substances that don't bother him today.

There are two choices. Turn around and avoid full-blown environmental illness with its attendant horrors, or deny that such a possibility as the things that happened to me could exist, and plunge out headlong into the vast unknown.

If you have begun to experience unusual physical and/or mental symptoms when either breathing or ingesting chemical substances, I hope you will take heed. Because of my own traumatic experience, I see a terrible urgency in your need to accept personal responsibility in this matter. To make an informed, deliberate, and reasonable choice. To run the other way as fast as you can go.

Had I done that—had I shied away from exposures when

they first began to make problems instead of tolerating each irritant until I couldn't stand it anymore—I might not have come so close to having the chemical monster devour me alive.

Group Three

These are the people whose reaction to chemicals is so subtle that they don't realize they're responding to them at all. We know now that I lived in this category for years before we had a clue as to what was wrong. Even later, when we knew that certain strong chemical exposures stopped my breathing, we didn't realize that much weaker concentrations of them were having less obvious effects on me. We simply didn't know that chemicals could be a problem when they existed at levels that were too low for my nose to detect.

This was really frustrating to my family. (Usually, in this sort of exposure, my responses were such that I wasn't aware of them; I'd become unreasonable and stubborn, but didn't know it.) My family could tell that something was wrong—maybe very wrong—but they couldn't identify the cause of the problem. They just knew that sometimes Mother's like this. Wait a while, and she'll be herself again.

Not until much further into my long illness did we come to understand, through reading some of the books listed in the appendix of this volume, that there's a tremendous potential for otherwise undetectable levels of pollutants to affect the thinking processes.

I'm still learning more about this from personal experience. When those who understand me best look at each other in a certain way and then go silent, I'm pretty safe in concluding that my thinking processes are being negatively impacted by chemicals I'm not aware of. My family wouldn't be aware of them either if it weren't for my "mental" response.

At the time, of course, I wonder what's wrong with my family. After all, I feel just fine, and here they are inferring that I'm off balance again. My brain is too befuddled by the allergens for me to realize that they really do have a reason to be passing those silent signals back and forth among them.

Now Where From Here?

It's almost seven years since the nutritionist first came to our house, and I'm down to the final rewriting of the final chapter of this book. I'm functioning reasonably well. Only once in a long while do I have an off day.

The nightmares and insomnia and phobias are gone. The disperceptions hardly ever raise their heads. The time lapses and suspended animation spells are rare indeed. The bloated feeling and gasiness come only when I cheat and eat sweets (which I can do occasionally now without serious repercussions.) The brain fag has cleared almost entirely. When I do get a bit of it, I know I've either cheated on sugar again or I've been exposed to low levels of chemicals in the air—levels I was not aware of at the time.

I'm advising others about nutrition now, and writing books for adults and having them published—things I'd never have dreamed seven years ago that I would ever do.

I have the satisfaction of feeling useful again, and some assurance that I'm not a burden to the people I love. I wake up in the morning thinking, "Well, let's see; what will I do first this morning? (It used to be "Do I have to get up? I'd rather just stay in bed.")

Seven years ago this month, our doctor told me, almost in so many words, "Go home and die." At the time, it was all I really wanted anyway. Today, I still look forward to the day when I'll wake up in heaven. But meanwhile, I'm also enjoying being here on earth.

From the bottom of my heart, I wish you the same or better.

For additional copies of this book, write to:
Bluebird Books,
Box 241, Dept. B
Unity, WI, 54488

As of the time of this printing, the price is $10.00 per copy, postpaid anywhere in the Continental USA. Pay by check or money order.

Credit cards not accepted. Sorry. Canadian orders remit in US funds, using an International Money Order, and add $2.00 per book for the extra postage needed to Canada.

Quantities of 10 or more to one address, for clubs, etc., $6.50 U.S. per book. Postpaid in the USA. Postage on 10 books to Canada, $6.00 extra.

Stores ordering for resale, contact the above address for wholesale pricing. (Standard discount given.) Thank you.

(Recommended retail price is $8.95)
These prices are subject to change.

APPENDIX

Recommended Reading

There is a huge selection of health books available today. Some of the most useful that we are acquainted with are listed below. We have noted some cautions after some of the titles. There may be some undesirable features in some of them that we have not issued a warning against. The fact that a book appears on this list does not mean that we endorse everything in it. We encourage you to read the last section in chapter ten of this book (A Word About Nutritionists, Etc.) and to fix in your mind some of the things to guard against . From there, you're on your own. We can not be responsible for the results of your reading.

1. Alternative Approach to Allergies By Dr. Theron Randolph, MD —a useful insight into just what allergy to chemicals can do to otherwise "normal" people. Dr. Randolph was the very first to discover this connection, late in the 1940s.

2. The E I Syndrome—An Rx for Environmental Illness By Dr. Sherry Rogers, MD —a wealth of information about environmental illness, including lists of places that chemicals hide. Also much info on food allergies. Only very little on detoxification.

—**WARNING**: she's very pro desensitization injections. In cases of chemical sensitivity, however, as she will tell you somewhere in the book, shots often lead to further sensitivity. So let the reader beware.

3. Brain Allergies By William Philpott, MD —the best single text we've found on the effects of food allergy on the functioning of the mind. He says little about allergy to chemicals in the air, but the effects are similar to those of allergy to foods. Excellent, but nothing on detoxification.

4. The Yeast Connection By William Crook, MD —very

useful discussion of candida yeast overgrowth and its effects on the body and on the mind. While candida isn't the sole player in the chemical story, it can be a major contributor.

—**WARNING**: a casual reading will leave you thinking that the drugs he discusses are the right route to recovery. In fact, those who use the drugs often end up with drug resistant strains of candida, which can be a nightmare of their own. But the information on the nature of candida overgrowth is of tremendous value. His questionnaire to determine whether you have a candida problem is excellent.

5. We Won't Let You Die! By Charlie Finch, with Dr. Jack Hinze, Pharmacist, Naturopath, and MD —autobiography of a professional commercial painter who almost lost his life as a result of the toxic effects of the paints, lacquers, etc., he used indiscriminately. There's a sizeable section by Dr. Hinze on the methods used for his recovery.

—**WARNING**: There's a heavy plug in here for Nature's Sunshine herbs. They're good, but so are several other brands, including Nature's Way and Nature's Herbs, which are available cheaper at the health food store. (Nature's Sunshine is multi-level, and more costly. Some of their dealers are honorable business persons, and some of them slander other products until you hardly know what to believe. So beware who you listen to.)

6. It's All in Your Head By Hal Huggins, DDS —a serious expose of the dangers of mercury-amalgam dental fillings in your teeth. Some people benefit greatly by having the mercury removed; others don't. A thorough and professional discussion of the problem. (Dr. Huggins is a dentist.)

7. Hypothyroidism: the Unsuspected Illness By Broda Barnes, MD —an in-depth discussion of the vitally important role of good thyroid function in maintaining overall health. Chemical sensitivity isn't mentioned in this book (it was written in 1976), but we now know that one of the imbalances that

allows sensitivity to develop is thyroid insufficiency.

—**WARNING**: His only remedy for thyroid insufficiency is to use the drug route. That wasn't so bad in 1976, when the book was written; they didn't have synthetic replacement thyroid hormone then. But even then, it would have been better to have gone the natural route, using ocean vegetation, flax seed oil, and vitamin B complex to restore normal function.

8. Remove the Thorn and God Will Heal By Bud Curtis — tells how the body gets toxic and how to cleanse it naturally.

9. Superimmunity for Kids By Leo Galland, MD —a thorough and excellent discussion of feeding children and young people to nourish their immune systems and thus prevent many of the major health problems plaguing our youth today.

10. Dr. Atkins' Health Revolution By Robert C Atkins, MD —first, he gives a clear description of the differences between "ordinary" medicine and "alternative" medicine. Then he describes "Complentary medicine" which embraces the best of both, and which is our preference. (We don't throw away the doctors just because we prefer natural methods wherever possible.)

—**WARNING**: he recommends a very high-protein diet, inferring that this is best for mankind. Since God gave Adam and Eve fruit to eat in Eden, we differ with his teaching on this point. We much prefer a diet that emphasizes fruits and vegetables, whole grains, and raw nuts and seeds, with a bit of meat sometimes, but not as the main course.

11. Your Body's Many Cries For Water By F. Batmanghelidj, MD —just might be the most important health book you'll ever read. A clear explanation of the body's need for water and our failure to fulfil that need, with the dire results of our neglect. Many illnesses, including serious ones, respond very nicely to nothing more than the consistent use of one-half ounce of water per pound of the person's present body weight

per day. All water is to be drunk between meals, with a special emphasis on using a generous portion about one half hour before you plan to eat.

DISCLAIMER: Neither the author nor the publisher takes any responsibility for the results you might obtain by implementing anything in any of the above volumes. It is your right to be informed and to decide for yourself what to do with your own body. But neither the author nor the publisher is accountable in any way for your decisions or for their outcome.

The Naturopathic Physician

As mentioned earlier in this book, the naturopathic physician is the most likely of all professional health care providers to have answers to chemical problems. He is accustomed to dealing with the whole person rather than a single gland or organ, and he is highly trained, having an education in health care equal to that of the ordinary medical doctor. He practices detoxification.

There are a few cautions to observe: as with all health care providers, there may be some aspects of the services offered that aren't desirable. So once again, read the last section of chapter twelve of this book to see what you might want to be alert to.

To locate the naturopathic physician nearest to you, you can contact the office below. If you choose to write, be forewarned that you won't get anything from them until you send them five dollars, which procures their national registry and directory. (1996 price.)

American Association of Naturopathic Physicians
2366 Eastlake Avenue East Suite 322
Seattle WA 98102
Phone: 206-323-7610 Voice mail only.

The Broda Barnes Foundation

For a free information packet on thyroid problems, call 203-261-2101. Be sure to request a list of participating physicians for your area.

Sources

ATTOGRAM. The company that invented the Caprol product that's at the heart of the Attogram Candida Purge. They also carry other products for intestinal cleansing. They sell both wholesale and retail. The following toll-free number is good in both Canada and the United States: 888-Fatigue (1-888-328-4483).

ACU-TROL. Located in Minneapolis-St. Paul, Monica carries a good selection of products for candida control. She sells by mail. Call her at 1-800-594-4675.

BIO-SAN LABS. This is the source of the MegaFood and Bio Metabolic supplements. (The two are identical.) For a referral to the store nearest you, call 1-800-848-2542. (See the section "Herbs and Vitamins Marry" in this book for a description of their products.)

NOW FOODS. This family owned company makes top quality supplements available at much lower prices than comparable products are. Call them at 1-630-545-9098 for a referral to a health food store near you that carries their line.

NUTRI-CHOICE. Located in Wisconsin, Nutri-Choice is a mail-order source for a large selection of supplements, including the Bio Metabolic line and the Attogram Candida Purge as well as many NOW Foods products. Most of the items they sell are discounted by about 35%. Their mail order catalog lists almost 500 different items. For a free catalog, call them at 1-715-223-3941. No Sunday calls.

SEDNA SPECIALTIES. A source of nutritional supplements and personal care products selected especially for those who are sensitive to chemicals. For a product list, call 1-800-223-0858. Mail order available.

PAT LEE. Source for antiparasitic herbs. Sells the book Remove the Thorn and God Will Heal. 1-800-888-1374.

Please note that neither the author nor the publisher can be held accountable for the results that you might obtain from using either products or advice from any of these sources.

Bonus Chapter

The following is from the forthcoming book, *Wellness: You Have to Start Somewhere*. It's by the same author as this book, and will be available through the same publisher. As a health minded reader, you'll find in it valuable information, much of which is overlooked in the major health publications.

Adrenal Exhaustion is Increasing

We often interview people who have health problems that the medical doctors can't help. These people usually have several health imbalances at the same time. Among them, adrenal weakness or even exhaustion is very common. The person with poor adrenal function will have several (though often not all) of the following symptoms:

1. He's tired most of the time, often more tired in the morning that he was when he went to bed. If he feels energetic at all during the day, it's in the late afternoon or early evening.
2. He gets lightheaded, dizzy, and/or fainty when he stands up after having been bent over for a while.
3. He feels exhausted (drained) when an emergency or a deadline is past. If his adrenal burnout is far advanced,

he'll be so rattled by an emergency or a deadline that he won't be able to cope with it at all. (Well-meaning friends often judge such folks as having spiritual problems, feeling that if someone goes to pieces under pressure, he isn't trusting the Lord.)

4. He gets shaky, feels faint or dizzy, has a headache, or becomes desperately hungry when he doesn't get his meals on time. He needs a snack to tide him over.
5. In the middle of the afternoon, he might suddenly feel either very hungry or very tired.
6. He might awaken at about three o'clock in the morning and not be able to go back to sleep. If he eats something, he can usually go back to sleep within a half hour.
7. Bright sunshine bothers his eyes, and he might have tinted glasses because he minds glare.
8. His blood pressure drops when he changes from prone to standing. To check, have the person lie down and relax for five minutes. Take his blood pressure while he's still down. Then have him stand and immediately take it again. Be sure that the cuff is on the same arm both times. For the standing reading, have the elbow at heart level. The systolic pressure (top number) should rise at least ten points when he stands. If it doesn't rise at all, suspect adrenal problems. If it drops, adrenal complications are even more likely.
9. He might have allergies or even asthma. While other irregularities, including immune system malfunction, are involved, allergies and asthma point directly to adrenal burnout—a point from which it's a long way back to normal.
10. He might experience apnea—the failure of the breathing reflex to function properly. This is especially likely to happen during the night, and he'll wake up gasping for breath.

Very few people have all of these symptoms. But those who do experience several of them should give serious consideration to the condition of their adrenal glands. They're our stress copers, and unfortunately the longer we continue to overstress them, the more likely we are to reach full-blown adrenal burnout.

The Solutions

Regenerating burned out adrenals takes many months—in some cases years. If you're already in actual burnout, you'll have to do a great many things very differently if you're ever to return to normal. Drastic diet changes, major lifestyle adjustments, and the taking of supplements are all involved. Otherwise, you'll keep on going downward.

If you've just reached the point where the adrenals are beginning to be overloaded, it's much easier to regain normal function. But if you don't take heed now, the day will likely come when you too are in full-blown adrenal burnout—and then it's a long way back.

Diet and Lifestyle Changes

1. *NO* sugar, honey, maple syrup, or dried fruit, nor any foods that contain any of them. Even the natural sweets whip the adrenals, making it much more difficult if not impossible for them to heal.
2. Absolutely *ZERO* caffeine. If anything is worse for the adrenals than sweets, it has to be caffeine. Avoid it totally, whether in coffee, tea, chocolate, or pain pills. (Read labels.)
3. Do *NOT* use any of the following herbs: ephedra, desert herb, ma haung, Brigham tea. These four names are all used for the same plant. It's a very effective adrenal stimulator—which is exactly what you don't need. Your adrenal glands are already overworked, and must relax and regenerate, not work even more. The above herbs make you more energetic temporarily. But in the

end they speed the day when your adrenals are totally exhausted, and then there's nothing left to stimulate. Moreover, when your adrenals are burned out, you can't work at all, no matter how hard you try to. (I know; I've been there.)

4. Take a five- to ten-minute rest break every two hours throughout the day. Assume whatever position is the most comfortable for you and relax as completely as you can. Concentrate on letting go of the tension in your body. It's especially helpful to relax the area around the eyes.
5. Divide your food into six small daily portions rather than three large meals. Because the adrenals are responsible for regulating blood sugar levels, less food at once makes less stress for them. (The pancreas makes the insulin, but the adrenals monitor its release into the blood stream.)
6. Eat mostly vegetables, whole grains (buckwheat, millet, brown rice, hominy, quinoa, amaranth, barley), dry beans, and raw nuts and seeds. Use a small amount of fruit. Meat should be very limited, for it places tremendous stress on both the pancreas and the adrenals. (Many vegetarians get hungry for meat once their adrenal function has been restored.)
7. Unload any responsibilities you can for a few months. Stressed adrenals hate pressure and deadlines. (When they're well, they help you to cope, and stress doesn't bother you. Strong adrenals are a major factor in staying calm.)
8. Use adrenal supporting supplements. The following section gives a realistic level to work up to if you're a normal sized adult and have serious adrenal problems. Smaller bodies need less, according to weight. Start slowly, taking one per day of each of perhaps half the recommended items. Add the others slowly, giving your system a chance to adjust to the new nutrients. When

you're taking some of each, then start to increase the quantities.

The Supplements

1. Pantothenic acid (vitamin B-5). 1,000 to 1,500 mg daily. Some folks do better yet on royal jelly, substituting one 1,000 mg capsule for each 500 mg of pantothenic acid.
2. Vitamin B Complex. Use a combination designed for stress. Aim for 100 mg daily of each of the major B-complex factors. Or use two to three per day of Bio Metabolic Nutrition's Balanced B-Complex. Its potencies are lower, but the absorption rate is much higher, and if often works where the ordinary types don't.
3. ADR-NL Combination from Nature's Way, or some other adrenal herbs combination. Take four to six per day. Some people get good results with an equal number of ginseng capsules per day instead.
4. Vitamin C, perferably Ester C. 2,000 to 3,000 mg per day.
5. Chromium picolinate. Need seems to range from 200 to 1,000 mcg per day. If taken toward evening, it might keep you awake. If so, don't take it after noon.
6. GLA (the initials stand for gammalinolenic acid) is essential for proper adrenal function. Start with one evening primrose seed oil capsule per day, and each week increase by one more per day until you're taking four per day. Then you can drop the primrose and go to one borage seed oil capsule daily. It's the same nutrient, and is more economical, but starting with a whole borage oil capsule can be quite a shock to the system. So go gradually, switching to borage after four weeks on primrose. Later, you might want to increase to two borage oil per day.
7. Seaweed. Either from three to six kelp capsules (not the tablets) daily, or one fourth to one half teaspoonful

of dulse liquid. Some folks use even more.

8. Adrenal glandular substance. Take according to the directions on the bottle. We don't usually find glandulars necessary, but some folks seem to benefit by using them.
9. Licorice root. We use this for men only, as it tends to increase the imbalance between estrogen and progesterone in women—an imbalance that's far too common anyhow. Men can use up to six capsules a day, or a rounded teaspoonful of the powder.

Adrenals and Allergies

When they're healthy and functioning as they ought to, the adrenals produce considerable quantities of anti-inflammatory substances. Allergies almost always indicate poor adrenal function. While other complications might be involved, it's surprising how often allergies improve or even disappear when adrenal health is restored.

Since allergies usually lead to more allergies—and more severe allergies as time goes on—it's wise to get to the root of the problem if possible. This is especially true when we consider the long term negative effects of allergy medications.

Adrenal Health and Body Toxicity

If you have the symptoms listed earlier in this chapter, and you don't get the help you had hoped for by following the recommendations given, then suspect body toxicity. The endocrine glands, including the adrenals, are very subject to the negative effects of stored toxins. If you have a toxic body, you'll have to address that before the adrenals will respond.

Notes

Notes